SIGNS AND SYMPTOMS IN PULMONARY MEDICINE

SIGNS AND SYMPTOMS IN PULMONARY MEDICINE

Edited by

FREDERICK L. GLAUSER, M.D.

Professor of Medicine
Chief, Pulmonary Division
Medical College of Virginia
Richmond, Virginia

12 contributors

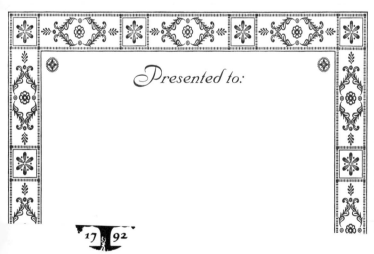

Presented to:

J. B. Lippincott Company • Philadelphia
London   Mexico City   New York   St. Louis   São Paulo   Sydney

Acquisitions Editor: Lisa A. Biello
Sponsoring Editor: Sanford J. Robinson
Manuscript Editor: Carol M. Kosik
Indexer: Julia Schwager
Designer: Sue Bishop
Production Supervisor: J. Corey Gray
Production Assistant: Barney Fernandes
Compositor: Tapsco
Printer/Binder: R. R. Donnelley & Sons Company

Library of Congress Cataloging in Publication Data
Main entry under title:

Signs and symptoms in pulmonary medicine.

  Bibliography: p.
  Includes index.
  1. Lungs—Diseases—Diagnosis. 2. Symptomatology.
I. Glauser, Frederick L. [DNLM: 1. Lung diseases—
Diagnosis. WF 600 S578]
RC756.S49   1983   616.2′4075   82-22862
ISBN 0-397-50544-2

The authors and publisher have exerted every effort to ensure that drug selection and dosage set forth in this text are in accord with current recommendations and practice at the time of publication. However, in view of ongoing research, changes in government regulations, and the constant flow of information relating to drug therapy and drug reactions, the reader is urged to check the package insert for each drug for any change in indications and dosage and for added warnings and precautions. This is particularly important when the recommended agent is a new or infrequently employed drug.

To Sue, who encouraged me to undertake this endeavor.

To Aaron and Brian for intermittently staying out of my hair.

CONTRIBUTORS

Kevin R. Cooper, M.D.
Assistant Professor of Medicine, Medical College of Virginia; Co-Medical Director, Respiratory Therapy Department and Pulmonary Function Laboratory, Richmond, Virginia

R. Paul Fairman, M.D.
Assistant Professor of Medicine, Medical College of Virginia; Director, General Medical Intensive Care Unit, Richmond, Virginia

Theodore Feinson, M.D.
Fellow, Pulmonary Disease, Medical College of Virginia–McGuire Veterans Administration Hospital, Richmond, Virginia

Frederick L. Glauser, M.D.
Professor of Medicine and Chief, Pulmonary Division, Medical College of Virginia, Richmond, Virginia

Albert "Mac" Marland, M.D.
Staff Physician, San Jose Hospital, San Jose, California

J. Eugene Millen
Pulmonary Physiologist, Associate Professor of Medicine, and Technical Director, Respiratory Intensive Care Unit, Medical College of Virginia, Richmond, Virginia; Technical Director, General Medical Intensive Care Unit, Pulmonary Function Laboratory, Respiratory Therapy Department, McGuire Veterans Administration Hospital, Richmond, Virginia

Calvin F. Morrow, M.D.
Assistant Professor of Medicine and Director, Pulmonary Function Laboratory and Respiratory Therapy Department, McGuire Veterans Administration Hospital, Richmond, Virginia

Orhan Muren, M.D.
Professor of Medicine, Co-Medical Director, Respiratory Therapy Department and Pulmonary Function Laboratory, and Director, Bronchoscopy, Medical College of Virginia, Richmond, Virginia

Barbara Phillips, M.D.
Instructor in Medicine, University of Kentucky Medical Center, Lexington, Kentucky

R. Crystal Polatty, M.D.
Fellow, Pulmonary Disease, Medical College of Virginia–McGuire Veterans Administration Hospital, Richmond, Virginia

Scott K. Radow, M.D.
Staff Physician, McGuire Clinic, Richmond, Virginia

James A. Thompson III, M.D.
Assistant Professor of Medicine, Medical College of Virginia; Chief, Pulmonary Section, McGuire Veterans Administration Hospital, Richmond, Virginia

PREFACE

"What limits people is that they don't have the . . . nerve
or imagination to star in their own movie, let alone
direct it."—From *Still Life with Woodpecker* by Tom Robbins

During the last decade, a plethora of excellent physiologically and clinically oriented books related to pulmonary disease have appeared directed toward the clinician. These books are traditional in the sense that they open with a general pulmonary physiology review and then discuss in detail specific disease processes. It would therefore seem inappropriate and unnecessary to add another book on pulmonary disease to the marketplace; however, we feel that *Signs and Symptoms in Pulmonary Medicine* may fill a niche which has been neglected or not appreciated by the traditional textbooks. The thrust and bulk of this book is toward symptoms and signs in pulmonary medicine as indicated by the title. It is intended to be a practical guide for medical students, practicing and graduate nurses with a special interest in respiratory patients, respiratory therapists, and specialized nurse practitioners.

To preserve consistency with the other textbooks in this series, our book is entitled *Signs and Symptoms in Pulmonary Medicine*, but a more logical title would be *Symptoms and Signs in Pulmonary Medicine* because in the clinical setting, the initial patient–medical personnel interface is usually the result of a specific complaint (e.g., the patient is suffering from a symptom or a group of symptoms). After obtaining these pertinent symptoms the physician or medical personnel performs a physical examination seeking specific signs of the disease process. The combinations of specific symptoms and signs leads to the formulation of an appropriate differential diagnosis.

The outline of this textbook has been established to mimic this clinical scenario. Chapters are based on symptoms and signs and not specific disease processes. Each chapter opens with an overview regarding mechanisms, physiology, differential diagnosis, and characteristics of the specific symptom or sign. This area can be read separately or in concert with the specific disease processes and their relation to the specific symptom under consideration.

The latter part of each chapter is organized as follows. An introduction defines the abbreviations and signs used in the table. A table consisting of 36 specific pulmonary diseases, groups of diseases, or syndromes with numbers assigned to each disease remaining constant throughout the text. For example, chronic bronchitis is consistently numbered 2 and sarcoidosis, 8. If a symptom or sign does not occur in a specific disease, that disease and its number will not appear in that particular chapter. In addition to the above, the table lists the presence and severity of each symptom and sign in relation to the specific disease. In the Comments column, additional information regarding the specific sign or symptom of the disease being considered may be found. If there are no comments next to a specific disease, there is nothing unique that needs to be mentioned.

To properly use this part of each chapter, the reader needs to assemble his patient's list of symptoms and signs and determine, through appropriate use of the table, in which disease processes these particular symptoms and signs are found. By working through each specific symptom and sign and the different disease processes, the reader should arrive at an appropriate differential diagnosis based on his patient's complaints and physical findings.

Chapter 22 lists all of the 36 disease entities considered and gives a brief overview of their common laboratory, chest radiographic, electrocardiographic, arterial blood gas, and pulmonary function abnormalities. This chapter is intended to acquaint the reader with each specific disease process.

Frederick L. Glauser, M.D.

ACKNOWLEDGMENTS

I would like to express my deep appreciation for the help of the pulmonary faculty at Medical College of Virginia and fellows who contributed their time and effort in preparing the individual chapters. In particular, I appreciate their patience and objectivity in tolerating the many revisions that went into each chapter. I would also like to thank Bonnie Deitrick, who spent long and grueling hours deciphering, transcribing, typing, retyping, and retyping this manuscript. Her speed and efficiency were unparalleled.

I would particularly like to thank R. Paul Fairman, M.D. for his valuable input into the design and layout in this book. His reviewing (and re-reviewing) of the entire book and specific chapters were invaluable.

Finally, I extend my appreciation to Ms. Suzette Stansell for her excellent artistry and patience.

CONTENTS

part I
SYMPTOMS

1 · DYSPNEA

R. PAUL FAIRMAN

FREDERICK L. GLAUSER

DEFINITION

Dyspnea is a subjective feeling of difficult, uncomfortable, or unpleasant breathing. The term is synonymous with "shortness of breath," the usual complaint offered by patients. Although unpleasant, dyspnea is not painful; it is rather an awareness of the need for increased respiratory effort. Most authorities believe that dyspnea is experienced when the perception of breathing is excessive for the level of activity. All individuals experience a form of dyspnea when performing maximal or near maximal exercise. Dyspnea must be differentiated from tachypnea and hyperpnea, which are objective findings of increased tidal volume and minute ventilation, respectively.

MECHANISMS

Knowledge of the sensors used and the integrated brain function necessary for awareness of dyspnea is still in its infancy. The following elements must be present to perceive dyspnea: a "sensing" organ or device, neurologic connections to the brain, integrating centers in the brain to process the essential information, and cortical connections to interpret the sensation.[1,2] Although many theories explaining dyspnea have been advanced, none have gained full acceptance.[3-7]

It has been proposed that stimulation of one of the following sensory devices either causes or contributes to dyspnea:

3

Irritant receptors in the lung parenchyma and airways

Juxta capillary receptors (J receptors) in the alveolar interstitium that respond to change in compliance[5]

Numerous muscle spindles found in the chest wall, joints, and costosternal junction that are less prevalent in the diaphragm and respond to stretch, movement, and proprioception

Carotid bodies or central nervous system respiratory centers activated through some combination of hypercapnea, hypoxemia, and acidosis[4]

Regardless of which sensing devices are used, the connecting pathways to the central nervous system are the vagal and phrenic nerves to the ascending reticular activating system in the brain stem. The higher cortical center connections responsible for the sensation of dyspnea reaching consciousness are unknown.

COMMON PHYSIOLOGICAL ABNORMALITIES FOUND IN PATIENTS WITH DYSPNEA

Patients experiencing dyspnea usually have severe airway obstruction (emphysema, bronchitis, asthma), a diffuse pulmonary parenchymal infiltrative process (pulmonary edema, interstitial fibrosis), or neuromuscular weakness (Guillain-Barré syndrome, myasthenia gravis). Patients with increased airway resistance have elevated functional residual capacity that causes lung hyperinflation, leading to shortening and inefficiency of inspiratory muscles. The increased effort necessary to sustain normal ventilation may be perceived by the patient as dyspnea. Some investigators feel that this sensation of dyspnea may be augmented by marked fluctuation in pleural pressures as is found in patients with both obstructive and restrictive diseases.[6]

Patients with infiltrative (restrictive) lung diseases usually have decreased lung volumes with noncompliant or stiff lungs. The stiffness may cause reflex stimulation of irritant, chest wall, or J receptors, leading to tachypnea and eventually dyspnea. Dyspnea in neuromuscular disease is related to decreased respiratory muscle strength and the patient's perception that his ventilation is inadequate for his activity.

DIFFERENTIAL DIAGNOSIS IN PATIENTS WITH DYSPNEA

Dyspnea is a common complaint of patients with both pulmonary and nonpulmonary disorders.

Nonpulmonary Causes of Dyspnea

Heart disease
  Left ventricular failure from any cause
  Aortic and mitral valvular disease (e.g., both stenosis and insufficiency)
  Cardiomyopathies
  Congenital heart defects
High cardiac output states (e.g., beriberi, hyperthyroidism, peripheral arteriovenous shunts)
Anemia
High altitude
Obesity
Anxiety
Excessive exercise
Deconditioning
Febrile states
Metabolic acidosis

Dyspnea with exercise or at rest. It is important to determine whether the onset of the dyspnea is sudden (bacterial or viral pneumonias, pulmonary emboli) or insidious (pulmonary emphysema, bronchitis). Everyone experiences a form of dyspnea with vigorous exercise, but when a disease process impairs respiratory capacity, less exercise is possible before dyspnea becomes evident. Dyspnea occurs at rest only with severely impaired respiratory capacity. In addition to measuring the extent and degree of dyspnea, the physician should elicit other symptoms and signs and relate them to the patients' complaints.

Positional dyspnea. Patients who experience orthopnea (dyspnea in the reclining position) usually show evidence of left ventricular dysfunction with resultant cardiogenic pulmonary edema. Most patients with chronic obstructive pulmonary disease (COPD) or advanced interstitial fibrosis have no or minimal orthopnea. Platypnea, defined as dyspnea on assuming the upright position, is sometimes found in patients with COPD, cirrhosis, and postpneumonectomy.[8-11] The etiology is unclear, but platypnea may be due to ventilation–perfusion mismatching or opening of a patent foramen ovale, which leads to hypoxemia (termed *orthodeoxia*) and subsequent positional dyspnea.

Paroxysmal nocturnal dyspnea. Awakening from sleep with shortness of breath is usually relieved by sitting up or walking around; patients with pulmonary disease do not experience true paroxysmal nocturnal dyspnea. A patient with pulmonary disease may occasionally complain of awakening at night and attribute it to dyspnea but careful questioning usually reveals that the patient wakes because of sputum accumulation and that the main problem is cough. During the coughing episodes, patients may experience dyspnea. This differentiation between true paroxysmal nocturnal dyspnea and coughing episodes is important because it allows the physician to decide whether the main problem is cardiac or pulmonary.[12]

DYSPNEA IN SPECIFIC PULMONARY DISEASES

The following table lists certain characteristics of dyspnea in relation to specific pulmonary diseases. A positive (+) sign signifies that dyspnea is the chief complaint in a specific disease; a positive/negative (±) sign means that dyspnea may be the chief complaint in a small percentage of patients; and a negative (−) sign means that dyspnea may be present but is not the chief complaint. Onset of dyspnea can be either insidious or sudden; the positive (+) sign indicates the type of onset for dyspnea in each disease. Special characteristics of dyspnea are found under the Comments heading. If no description appears in this column, no special features of dyspnea occur in the specific disease being considered.

| Disease | Chief complaint of dyspnea | Onset | | Comments |
		Insid-ious	Sud-den	
Obstructive lung disease				
Common				
1. Emphysema	+	+	−	Dyspnea may severely limit the patient's activities; platypnea is found in a small percentage of these patients; orthopnea and paroxysmal nocturnal dyspnea are absent.
2. Chronic bronchitis	−	+	−	
3. Asthma	−	−	+	Dyspnea may be a main complaint depending on the severity of the attack; dyspnea disappears between attacks.

Disease	Chief complaint of dyspnea	Onset Insid-ious	Onset Sud-den	Comments
Uncommon				
4. Bronchiectasis	−	+	−	Severity of dyspnea increases when associated with lower respiratory tract infections.
5. Cystic fibrosis	−	+	−	Similar to bronchiectasis.
Restrictive lung disease				
Common				
7. Interstitial fibrosis	+	+	−	Dyspnea is progressive in nature, noted first with exercise and later at rest; many patients are limited in their activities.
8. Sarcoidosis	±	+	−	Dyspnea is relatively mild; in a small percentage of patients, progressive pulmonary involvement eventuates in dyspnea at rest.
9. Pulmonary edema	+	+	+	Patients with severe pulmonary edema suffer air hunger and a feeling of suffocation. Pulmonary edema of cardiac origin is associated with orthopnea and paroxysmal nocturnal dyspnea.
10. Thoracic cage deformities and abnormalities	±	+	−	
11. Neuromuscular disorders	±	+	+	
12. Inhalational or occupational pulmonary diseases	±	+	+	Patients with silicosis or coal miner's pneumoconiosis experience dyspnea of insidious onset whereas those acutely exposed to toxic fumes (chlorine, nitrogen dioxide, etc.) have the explosive onset of dyspnea.

Disease	Chief complaint of dyspnea	Onset		Comments
		Insidious	Sudden	
Uncommon				
13. Hypersensitivity pneumonitis	+	+	+	Dyspnea classically occurs 6–8 hr after exposure to the offending agent; patients experience air hunger and chest tightness. In the chronic form of this disease, dyspnea may be both progressive and insidious.
14. Goodpasture's syndrome	−	+	+	
15. Idiopathic pulmonary hemosiderosis	+	+	−	
16. Eosinophilic granuloma	+	+	−	These patients are prone to pneumothorax, which may account for a sudden increase in the severity of dyspnea.
Pulmonary vascular disease				
Common				
17. Acute pulmonary embolism	+	+	−	
Uncommon				
18. Sickle cell disease	−	+	−	Dyspnea may be progressive in patients with multiple *in situ* vascular thrombi and cor pulmonale.
19. Recurrent pulmonary thromboembolism	+	+	−	
20. Primary pulmonary hypertension	+	+	−	
21. Pulmonary veno-occlusive disease	+	+	−	

Disease	Chief complaint of dyspnea	Onset Insid- ious	Onset Sud- den	Comments
Tumors of the lung, pleura, and mediastinum				
Common				
22. Carcinoma of the lung	–	+	–	Sudden increase in shortness of breath occasionally occurs secondary to acute obstructive atelectasis or with obstructive pneumonia.
23. Metastatic carcinoma of the lung	–	+	–	Degree of dyspnea depends on the mass of lung replaced by the tumor and the extent of pleural implants or effusions; patients with lymphangitic spread of carcinoma may suffer severe dyspnea.
Uncommon				
25. Bronchial adenomas	–	+	±	Dyspnea may occur suddenly in acute airway obstruction with lobar atelectasis.
Infectious disease of the lung				
Common				
26. Bacterial, mycoplasmal, and rickettsial pneumonias	±	+	+	Dyspnea is a major complaint and depends on the extent of lung involvement, the presence of any underlying lung disease, and involvement of the pleura (e.g., pleural effusion).
27. Viral pneumonias	–	+	+	
28. Lung abscesses	–	+	–	

Disease	Chief complaint of dyspnea	Onset Insidious	Onset Sudden	Comments
29. Tuberculosis	−	+	−	Dyspnea may be secondary to pleural effusions, pulmonary involvement, or an associated anemia.
Uncommon				
30. Atypical tuberculosis	−	+	−	These patients usually have a history of underlying lung disease or chronic cavitation; dyspnea may therefore be present and worsen as the disease progresses.
31. *Actinomyces* and *Nocardia*	−	+	+	
32. Mycoses	−	+	+	
Miscellaneous				
33. Aspiration lung diseases	±	+	+	Dyspnea may be severe and sudden in onset depending on the type of material aspirated and the extent of lung involvement.
34. Pulmonary alveolar proteinosis	−	+	−	
35. Wegener's granulomatosis, its variants, and other vasculitides	−	+	−	

REFERENCES

1. Campbell EJM: Evaluation of dyspnea: Understanding breathlessness. Trans Med Soc Lond 92:13, 1975–1976
2. Campbell EJM: The relationship of the sensation of breathlessness to the act of breathing. In Howell BL, Campbell EJM (eds): Breathlessness, p 55. Oxford, Blackwell Scientific Publications, 1966

3. Christie RV: Dyspnea in relation to the visco-elastic properties of the lung. Proc R Soc Med (London) 46:481, 1954

4. Comroe JH Jr: Some theories of the mechanisms of dyspnea. In Howell BL, Campbell EJM (eds): Breathlessness, p 1. Oxford, Blackwell Scientific Publications, 1966

5. Paintal AS: Vagal sensory receptors and the reflex effects. Physiol Rev 53:159, 1973

6. O'Connel JM, Campbell AH: Respiratory mechanics and airway obstruction associated with respiratory dyspnea. Thorax 31:669, 1976

7. Moisan TC, Chandrasekhar AJ, Sharpe JT: Asynchronous breathing: Possible etiology for dyspnea in a patient with normal lungs. Chest 75:624, 1979

8. Ault M, Robin ED: Platypnea (diffuse zone I phenomenon). N Engl J Med 281:1347, 1969

9. Begin R: Platypnea after pneumonectomy. N Engl J Med 293:342, 1975

10. Robin ED, Lamen D, Horne BR et al: Platypnea related to orthodeoxia caused by true vascular lung shunts. N Engl J Med 294:941, 1976

11. Kahn F, Pareka A: Reversible platypnea and orthodeoxia following recovery from adult respiratory distress syndrome. Chest 75:526, 1979

12. Raffin TA, Theodore J: Separating cardiac from pulmonary dyspnea. JAMA 238:206, 1977

2 · COUGH

ORHAN MUREN

DEFINITION

Cough is a sudden and explosive forcing of air through the glottis to expel mucus or other material from the tracheal–bronchial tree. Coughing protects the lower respiratory tract against aspiration and provides a means of clearing retained secretions or foreign material from major airways. It is a cardinal manifestation in many chest diseases.

MECHANISMS

Coughing is basically a reflex act arising from stimulation of cough or irritant receptors located in the pharynx, larynx, trachea, and large bronchi. It can also be initiated and suppressed voluntarily. Coughing may occur following stimulation of receptors in the lung and visceral pleura. The stimuli are transmitted by branches of the glossopharyngeal and vagus nerves to the medullary cough center. The efferent arc consists of the recurrent laryngeal nerve and spinal nerves, which when stimulated cause glottic closure and contractions of the chest and abdominal muscles, respectively.[1-3]

Coughing can be divided into three phases: a deep inspiration; closure of the glottis with relaxation of the diaphragm and contraction of the muscles of expiration; and opening of the glottis, which causes a sudden blast of air through the lobar and mainstem bronchi and trachea and pushes any particulate substance or retained secretions toward the mouth. Contraction of the expiratory muscles against a closed glottis generates very high intrathoracic pressures (up to 300 mm Hg) that result in narrowing of the tracheal diameter. Large pressure gradients are produced between the bronchi and the atmosphere when the glottis opens, and this produces tracheal flow rates close to the speed of sound when associated with tracheal narrowing. The efficacy of a cough depends on the depth of the preceding inspiration and the degree of dynamic compression of the airways.[4]

Maximal expiratory flow rates depend on a number of factors including the amount of force generated by the contracting expiratory muscles, the intrinsic lung elastic recoil pressure, and airway resistance. In addition, the location of airway compression, the equal pressure point (EPP), is critical (Fig. 2–1).[5,6]

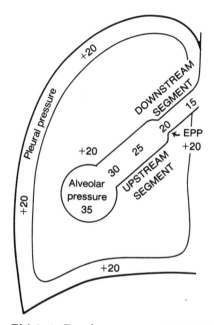

Fig. 2–1. Equal pressure point (EPP). Pleural pressures rise as muscular force is increased and transmitted to the alveoli. The driving pressure for flow (alveolar pressure, +35 cm H_2O) will equal the sum of pleural (+20 cm H_2O) and elastic recoil pressures (15 cm H_2O). During forced expiration, airway resistance decreases pressure along the airway; the pressure inside the airway lumen becomes equal to the pressure outside the airway (pleural pressure) as elastic recoil pressure of the lungs dissipates; this is called the *equal pressure point* or EPP. The airway between the EPP and the alveolus is termed the *upstream segment* and that from EPP to the mouth, the *downstream segment*.

At large lung volumes, elastic recoil pressure is high and no EPP develops. Air flow is effort dependent. At smaller lung volumes, elastic recoil pressure is decreased, and the EPP develops within the chest as dynamic airway compression occurs. Flow becomes effort independent. At the smallest lung volumes (e.g., near residual volume), the EPP moves as far upstream as possible, the furthest upstream movement being the level of the segmental bronchi in normal people. The EPP moves closer to the alveolus in patients with emphysema, impairing the efficacy of the cough by compression of the airways.

ETIOLOGY

Cough is initiated by inflammatory, chemical, mechanical, and thermal stimulation of the appropriate receptors. Mucosal edema with excessive tracheobronchial secretions secondary to acute viral laryngotracheal bronchitis, chronic bronchitis, and pneumonias are examples of inflammatory stimuli.[1] Chemical and thermal stimulation occur with the inhalation of irritant gases (e.g., cigarette smoke) and very hot or cold air.[7,8] Mechanical stimulation can arise from compression of the airways secondary to lung neoplasm, mediastinal tumor, or aortic aneurysm. The sudden onset of cough may signal the presence of a foreign body causing partial airway obstruction. Postnasal drip is a common but often unrecognized form of mechanical stimulation leading to coughing.[9,10]

A dry nonproductive cough is a common complaint of patients with stiff (e.g., noncompliant) lungs secondary to diffuse interstitial pneumonitis, fibrosis, or pulmonary edema. A dry, recurrent cough may be caused by wax or foreign bodies in the external auditory meatus due to stimulation of Arnold's nerve, a branch of the vagus. Some patients with asthma do not wheeze but complain of a chronic cough that awakens them from sleep.[11-13]

Some patients complain of a longstanding dry, nonproductive cough associated with throat clearing. No underlying disease can be found in these patients; they are characteristically nervous, and the cough is a nervous habit.

DIAGNOSTIC ASSESSMENT

A careful history and physical examination constitute the most important first step in the evaluation of cough. The physician must determine whether the patient's cough is acute or chronic, productive of sputum, and associated with other symptoms. Women tend to swallow sputum, and this may lead to the erroneous impression that the cough is nonproductive. Abnormal findings on examination of the chest and ear, nose, and throat should be sought. The chest x-ray must be carefully evaluated.

COMPLICATIONS

Tussive syncope occurs in cigarette-smoking men who experience paroxysms of uncontrollable coughing. The syncope is probably related to an acute fall in cardiac output due to reduced venous return to the heart resulting from the very high intrathoracic pressures generated. Rib fractures may occur if coughing is strenuous, even in normal people; however, the possibility of pathologic fractures such as those that occur with malignant lesions and osteoporosis should be considered. Finally, a subpleural bleb may rupture and produce a pneumothorax during violent coughing spells.

COUGH IN SPECIFIC PULMONARY DISEASES

The following table lists certain characteristics of cough in relation to specific pulmonary diseases. A positive (+) sign signifies that cough is *always* the chief complaint; a positive/negative (±) sign indicates that cough *may* be the chief complaint; and a negative (−) sign means that cough may be present but *is not* the chief complaint. The severity of cough is classified as follows: 1 is mild—occasional during the day and does not awaken patients at night; 2 is moderate—persistent during the day and occasionally awakening patients at night; and 3 is severe—paroxysms of cough are uncontrollable and awaken patients at night.

Disease	Chief complaint of cough	Severity	Comments
Obstructive lung disease			
Common			
2. Chronic bronchitis	+	2–3	Cough varies from a smoker's cough, which is dry, nonproductive, and usually worse in in the morning, to a persistent, debilitating cough associated with sputum production. Many patients smoke cigarettes to induce coughing and sputum production on arising in the morning.
3. Asthma	±	1–2	Coughing is usually associated with diffuse wheezing. Coughing may produce mucoid and tenacious sputum toward the end of an attack; however, a chronic nocturnal cough may be the only complaint in a certain subset of patients.
Uncommon			
4. Bronchiectasis	+	2–3	Cough is productive of copious, purulent, and foul-smelling sputum (see Chap. 3).

Disease	Chief complaint of cough	Severity	Comments
5. Cystic fibrosis	+	2–3	Similar to bronchiectasis.
6. Upper airway obstruction	±	1–3	Foreign body aspiration induces coughing. High-grade tracheal obstruction is associated with signs of asphyxiation. A nonproductive cough and a localized wheeze may be noted if a foreign body lodges in the lower airway. A "brassy" cough may be present in patients with upper airway obstruction due to tracheal or large airway tumors.

Restrictive lung disease
Common

Disease	Chief complaint of cough	Severity	Comments
7. Interstitial fibrosis	–	1	Cough is usually mild, nonproductive, but persistent; it is provoked by a deep inspiration in advanced interstitial fibrosis of any cause.
8. Sarcoidosis	–	1	Cough is nonproductive when present; a productive cough may occur due to complicating bronchitis or pneumonia in end-stage disease.
9. Pulmonary edema	–	1–3	Patients with cardiogenic pulmonary edema may complain of a nocturnal cough that awakens them in the early morning and is relieved by sitting upright. Cough is productive of frothy, pink sputum in a small percentage of patients with severe pulmonary edema. Cough is less common in patients with noncardiogenic pulmonary edema.
12. Occupational or inhalational pulmonary diseases	–	1–3	Cough that is dry or productive of mucoid sputum can be seen in a variety of occupational lung diseases. Examples include coal miner's pneumoconiosis, byssinosis, and grain worker's lung.

Disease	Chief complaint of cough	Sever-ity	Comments
Uncommon			
13. Hypersensitivity pneumonitis	–	2–3	Cough is common and nonproductive in acute hypersensitivity pneumonitis; it is less common in the subacute and chronic forms of this disease.
14. Goodpasture's syndrome	–	1–2	Cough is common and may be dry or productive of bloody sputum.
15. Idiopathic pulmonary hemosiderosis	–	1–2	Similar to Goodpasture's syndrome.
16. Eosinophilic granuloma	–	1–2	Cough is nonproductive.
Pulmonary vascular disease			
Common			
15. Acute pulmonary embolism	–	1–2	Approximately 50% of these patients complain of a cough that may be productive of bloody sputum.
Tumors of the lung, pleura, and mediastinum			
Common			
22. Carcinoma of the lung	+	1–3	The onset of a new cough or change in the character of an existing cough is a common complaint. Cough may be either nonproductive or productive depending on the location of the tumor.
24. Malignant mesothelioma	–	1	A dry, nonproductive cough is common.
Uncommon			
25. Bronchial adenoma	–	1–2	Cough is uncommon unless the patient develops airway obstruction with distal pneumonitis; the cough may then be productive.

Disease	Chief complaint of cough	Severity	Comments
Infectious diseases of the lung			
Common			
26. Bacterial, mycoplasmal, and rickettsial pneumonia	±	1–3	Cough productive of purulent sputum is a common complaint in patients with bacterial pneumonias. A recurrent hacking cough persisting after the successful treatment of the pneumonia is characteristic of mycoplasma pneumonia. A dry, nonproductive cough is common in rickettsial pneumonias.
27. Viral pneumonias	−	1–2	Cough is usually dry but may produce mucoid sputum.
28. Lung abscesses	±	2–3	Cough is common with large lung abscesses and may produce prodigious amounts of purulent, foul-smelling sputum. The cough tends to be persistent but can be paroxysmal.
29. Tuberculosis	±	1–3	Patients who cough and produce sputum are highly infective.
Uncommon			
30. Atypical tuberculosis	−	1–3	
31. *Actinomyces* and *Nocardia*	−	1–3	
32. Mycoses	−	1–3	
33. Aspiration lung disease	±	1–3	A persistent paroxysmal cough may occur with aspiration of both solid and liquid material.
35. Wegener's granulomatosis, its variants, and other vasculitides	−	1–2	

REFERENCES

1. Langlands J: The dynamics of cough in health and in chronic bronchitis. Thorax 22:88, 1967
2. Jones JG, Clarke SW: Dynamics of cough. Br J Anaesth 57:280, 1970
3. Irwin RS, Rosen MJ, Braman SS: Cough: A comprehensive review. Arch Intern Med 137:1186, 1977
4. Lawson TV, Harris RS: Assessment of the mechanical efficiency of coughing in healthy young adults. Clin Sci 33:209, 1967
5. Knudson RJ, Mead J, Knudson DE: Contribution of airway collapse to supramaximal expiratory flows. J Appl Physiol 36:653, 1974
6. Smaldone GC, Itoh H, Swift DL et al: Effect of flow-limiting segments and cough on particle desposition and mucociliary clearance in the lung. Am Rev Respir Dis 120:747, 1979
7. Loudon RG, Brown LC, Hurst SK: Cough frequency in a group of males. Arch Environ Health 11:372, 1965
8. Loudon RG: Smoking and cough frequency. Am Rev Respir Dis 114:1033, 1976
9. Irwin RS, Pratter MR: Postnasal drip and cough. Clin Notes Respir Dis 18:11, 1980
10. Letter to the Editor: Does postnasal drip cause cough? Clin Notes Respir Dis 18:7, 1979
11. Corrao WM, Bramam SS, Irwin RS: Chronic cough as the sole presenting manifestation of bronchial asthma. N Engl J Med 300:633, 1979
12. Loudon RG, Rapyrik N, Walsh JK et al: Coughing during sleep. Clin Res 28:781A, 1980
13. Glauser FL: Variant asthma. Ann Allergy 30:457, 1972

3 · SPUTUM PRODUCTION

JAMES A. THOMPSON III

ORHAN MUREN

DEFINITION

Sputum is an aggregation of secretions from the tracheobronchial tree, mouth, pharynx (saliva), nose, and sinuses. Phlegm refers to lung and tracheobronchial tree secretions.

CHARACTERISTICS

In healthy individuals, the daily volume of sputum produced is small and normally does not give rise to coughing or expectoration; therefore, the general rule is that any sputum production is abnormal. A patient may swallow large amounts of sputum unconsciously and thus give a negative history for sputum production. Furthermore, coughing does not necessarily indicate sputum production because the patient may have a dry, nonproductive cough (see Chap. 2); conversely, mucus can be secreted in large amounts without coughing.[1-3]

MECHANISMS

The respiratory system is the major interface between the external environment and the body's internal milieu. Mucus flow is one of the primary mechanisms for clearance of inhaled particulate material.[4-7] The volume of secretions cleared daily may approach 100 ml in a healthy adult; however, these secretions are swallowed and rarely expectorated. Normal tracheobronchial fluid is composed of secretions from the mucus glands and goblet cells and transudations from serum (Fig. 3–1). Sputum constituents include exfoliated epithelial cells, glycoproteins, bacteriostatic proteins (primarily lysozymes), lactoferrin, secretory IgA, and serum proteins (primarily albumin).[2,8–10] This material constitutes the mucus blanket that overlies the cilia. The mucus blanket helps remove foreign particles, assists in killing bacteria, and protects the respiratory epithelium from water loss. The above mechanisms help keep normal secretions bacteria free.

During acute or chronic inflammation and irritation or in certain pathologic states, the volume of sputum may increase due to excessive production of mucus and serous secretions. This results in a mucoid sputum that is clear, colorless, thin, and elastic in consistency. Purulent sputum is yellow–green and opaque; it is usually more viscous and less elastic than mucoid sputum. The yellow–green color results from an enzyme (myeloperoxidase) liberated during cellular breakdown of leukocytes.[11] It is therefore possible

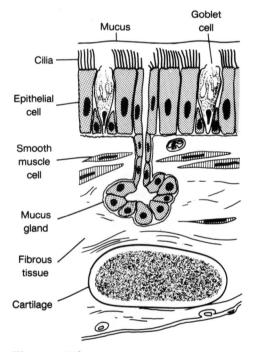

Fig. 3–1. Schematic cross-section of a large bronchus showing the relationships of the goblet cells and the mucus glands to the mucus lining layer. Specialized epithelial cells equipped with cilia line the lumenal border.

that the yellow–green color may be due to retained or stagnant secretions and not to an acute infection as generally accepted.

DIFFERENTIAL DIAGNOSIS

Characterization of sputum is important in assessing the type and severity of pulmonary disease and should include the following:

1. The amount of sputum produced daily
2. The color—clear, white (mucoid), yellow–green (purulent), or a combination
3. The presence of blood
4. The odor
5. Whether the patient feels that the sputum originates from a particular region of the lung
6. The presence of bronchial casts or stones

Extremely thick and tenacious sputum may be produced in patients with cystic fibrosis and asthma or in those suffering from dehydration. Massive sputum production (bronchorrhea) can be seen in patients with alveolar cell carcinoma, bronchitis, asthma, lung abscess, or empyema with bronchial communication.[12]

Yellow or bile-stained sputum is rarely produced by jaundiced patients. Amebic liver abscesses may rupture through the diaphragm into the lung, producing a bile-colored or "anchovy paste" sputum.

A red or reddish brown color suggests the presence of blood (Chap. 5), but a reddish tint can also result from aerosolized bronchodilators. *Serratia marcescens* pneumonia may rarely give rise to a reddish sputum. Reddish sputum secondary to inhalation of iron oxide pigment can be found in glass sanders. A gray or black discoloration occurs in sputum of coal miners, smokers, acute smoke inhalation victims, and in some patients with pulmonary mucormycosis. Blue sputum has been noted in copper miners. Additional discolorations may result from contamination with food or liquid pigments. Expectoration of chalky material or small stones is characteristic of broncholithiasis. The broncholiths are usually due to prior infections with tuberculosis, histoplasmosis, or coccidioidomycosis.

Patients with chronic sinusitis may have a nocturnal postnasal drip with a resultant early morning cough productive of mucopurulent sputum. Lipoid pneumonia may be due to inhalation or aspiration of mineral, vegetable, or animal oils. Cough and dyspnea occur, and there may be marked sputum production. A history of oily nose drop use and appropriate staining of the sputum is usually necessary for diagnosis.

Pulmonary diseases associated with parasites are uncommon in the United States; however, several parasitic infections give rise to chronic sputum production, including paragonimiasis, schistosomiasis, echinococcus, and amebiasis.

SPUTUM PRODUCTION IN SPECIFIC PULMONARY DISEASES

The following table lists characteristics of sputum production in relation to the specific pulmonary diseases. A positive (+) sign signifies that sputum production is the chief complaint; a positive/negative (±) sign indicates that in a certain percentage of patients, sputum production *may* be the chief complaint; and a negative (−) sign means that sputum production may be present but *is not* the chief complaint. The severity of sputum production is classified as follows: 1 is mild—less than ¼ cup/day; 2 is moderate—¼ cup/day; and 3 is severe—more than ¼ cup/day.

Disease	Chief complaint of sputum production	Severity	Comments
Obstructive lung disease			
Common			
2. Chronic bronchitis	+	1–3	Sputum is usually mucoid and may turn purulent during acute exacerbations or superimposed infections.
3. Asthma	−	1–3	Sputum production is characteristically scant during mild to moderate asthma attacks. The sputum becomes mucoid and tenacious, resulting in bronchial mucus plugging during severe attacks. Purulent sputum indicates either the presence of stasis or a secondary bacterial or viral infection.

Disease	Chief complaint of sputum production	Severity	Comments
Uncommon			
4. Bronchiectasis	+	2–3	The sputum is similar to that found in patients with chronic bronchitis; however, sputum production becomes more copious and purulent as the disease progresses. The amount of sputum varies considerably but may be voluminous. Increased production is most likely during the winter. Classically, collected sputum eventually separates into three layers. The lower layer is composed of thick purulent material, the middle layer consists of mucus mixed with purulent material, and the thin top layer is mucus. Concomitant chronic sinusitis is common in patients with bronchiectasis.
5. Cystic fibrosis	+	2–3	Sputum is characteristically thick, mucoid, and tenacious and may be malodorous. Chronic bronchial obstruction due to large mucus plugs with secondary parenchymal lung infections is common.
6. Upper airway obstruction	–	1	Sputum production is uncommon but may be due to mucus stasis occurring behind a high-grade obstruction.

Disease	Chief complaint of sputum production	Severity	Comments
Restrictive lung disease			
Common			
9. Pulmonary edema	—	1–3	Patients with florid pulmonary edema may produce thin, foamy, pinkish sputum. This liquid is not true sputum but rather results from transudation of plasma across the alveolar capillary membrane into the alveoli. This liquid may move up the tracheobronchial tree.
12. Inhalational or occupational pulmonary disease	—	1–3	Sputum production can follow the inhalation of noxious substances that eventuate in either acute or chronic bronchitis. Certain noxious gases may be responsible for sputum production secondary to pulmonary edema.
Tumors of the lung, pleura, and mediastinum			
Common			
22. Carcinoma of the lung	—	1–2	Sputum production is unusual in bronchogenic carcinoma unless there is associated chronic bronchitis or tumor causes airway obstruction resulting in distal pneumonia. A patient with alveolar cell carcinoma may occasionally produce copious watery sputum.
Uncommon			
25. Bronchial adenoma	—	1–2	Sputum production is usually due to obstructive pneumonias.

Disease	Chief complaint of sputum production	Severity	Comments
Infectious diseases of the lung			
Common			
26. Bacterial, mycoplasmal, and rickettsial pneumonias	±	2–3	Bacterial pneumonias must always be considered when the patient has a cough productive of purulent sputum. Onset of sputum production is relatively sudden.
28. Lung abscesses	+	2–3	Many patients with lung abscesses produce a foul-smelling, purulent sputum. Sudden onset of copious sputum production is usually associated with drainage of the cavity.
29. Tuberculosis	±	1–3	Sputum production is common and may be associated with hemoptysis (see Chap. 5).
Uncommon			
30. Atypical tuberculosis	±	1–3	
31. *Actinomyces* and *Nocardia*		1–2	
32. Mycoses	±	1–3	Sputum production is common in patients with mycotic pneumonias. Patients with aspergillus fungus balls (*aspergillomas*) usually complain of chronic sputum production that is often blood streaked (see Chap. 5).
Miscellaneous			
33. Aspiration lung disease	–	1–2	Aspiration of gastric contents results in sputum production due to a secondary pneumonia, bronchitis, bronchiectasis, or loss of alveolar capillary membrane integrity.

Disease	Chief complaint of sputum production	Severity	Comments
35. Wegener's granulomatosis, its variants, and other vasculitides	–	1–2	Cough productive of purulent or blood-tinged sputum may be seen with necrotic lesions. In addition, nasal drainage may be confused with sputum.

REFERENCES

1. Dulfano M: Sputum: Fundamental and Clinical Pathology. Springfield, IL, Charles C Thomas, 1973
2. Yeager H, Jr: Tracheobronchial secretions. Am J Med 50:4, 1971
3. Clifford R: The Sputum: Its Examination and Clinical Significances. New York, Macmillan, 1932
4. Osmundson T, Kilburn KH: Mucociliary clearance rates at various levels in dog lungs. Am Rev Respir Dis 102:388, 1970
5. Carson S, Goldhamer R, Carpenter R: Mucous transport in the respiratory tract. Symposium on Structure, Function and Measurement of Respiratory Cilia. Am Rev Respir Dis 93:86, 1966
6. Reid L: Sputum and mucociliary clearance mechanisms. Postgrad Med J 52:183, 1976
7. Green GM, Jakab GJ, Low RB et al: Defense mechanism of the respiratory membrane. Am Rev Respir Dis 115:479, 1977
8. Chodosh S, Baigelman W, Pizzuto D: Examining sputum. Am Fam Phys, 12, No. 3:116, 1975
9. Chodosh S: Examination of sputum cells. N Engl J Med 282:854, 1970
10. Epstein RL: Constituents of sputum: A simple method. Ann Intern Med 77:259, 1972
11. Robertson AJ: Green sputum. Lancet 1:12–15, 1952
12. Lopez V, Charman I, Keal E et al: Bronchorrhoea. Thorax 30:624, 1975

4 · CHEST PAIN

ORHAN MUREN

DEFINITION

Chest pain can be divided into two types: pleuritic and nonpleuritic. Pleuritic chest pain is usually located posteriorly or laterally, is sharp and stabbing in nature, is worsened by deep breathing and coughing, and is relieved by breath holding or "splinting" the affected side of the chest. Pain arises from the chest wall, muscles, ribs, parietal pleura, large airways, diaphragm and mediastinal structures, and intercostal nerves.

Nonpleuritic chest pain is usually located centrally, is constant and aching or boring in nature, and may radiate. It is most often nonpulmonary in origin although it is associated with certain pulmonary diseases.

MECHANISMS AND DIFFERENTIAL DIAGNOSIS

Chest pain is one of the most common complaints in clinical medicine. Many patients fear their chest pain is due to serious organic lung or heart disease. Correct diagnosis depends on an extensive physical examination, special studies, a history detailing the site and radiation, nature and duration, and aggravating factors related to the pain.

Pleuritic Chest Pain

Pleural effusion due to pulmonary infections, pulmonary embolism, connective tissue disorders, malignancies, or subdiaphragmatic inflammation causes pleuritic chest pain. Trichinosis of the chest wall muscles can produce pleuritic-type chest pain. The patients usually develop periorbital and generalized edema with peripheral blood eosinophilia. Pleuritic chest pain is a common complaint of patients with spontaneous pneumothorax, whereas chest pain and a crunching sound over the heart, audible on auscultation, are common findings in patients with pneumomediastinum.[1,2]

Nonpleuritic Chest Pain

Cardiac. Myocardial ischemia occurs when myocardial oxygen demands cannot be met by coronary blood flow. In patients with coronary artery disease, blood flow is limited by high-grade vascular obstruction. Afferent visceral nerve fibers are stimulated during myocardial ischemia, but the cerebral cortex cannot localize these signals as being myocardial in origin because the nervous impulses enter the spinal cord at levels T_1 to T_4, stimulating sensory pathways from other somatic sites.

Three different ischemic syndromes are recognized as angina of effort, acute coronary insufficiency or unstable angina, and myocardial infarction.[3] Myocardial ischemia generally produces squeezing or viselike substernal pain that radiates toward the axillae and down the inner sides of the arms. The left arm is involved more often than the right. Radiation to the epigastrium, neck, jaw, tongue, teeth, thumb, or mastoid may occur with or without substernal chest discomfort. Patients commonly express their pain with a clenched fist placed on the sternum to indicate both the site and the character of the sensation (the Levine sign).

Substernal chest pain experienced during exertion and relieved by rest was described by Heberdon (in 1768) as "angina pectoris." Attacks typically last only a few minutes and are relieved with nitroglycerin or rest. The pain may be provoked by meals, cold weather, sympathetic overreactivity as exemplified by emotional disturbance, or REM (rapid eye movement) sleep associated with dreaming. A stabbing pain lasting 1 or 2 seconds or chest pain following cessation of physical exercise is usually not anginal. Variant or Prinzmetal's angina is caused by spasm of normal or atherosclerotic coronary vessels; it occurs at rest and is associated with characteristic electrocardiographic changes.[4]

Coronary insufficiency or unstable angina pectoris should be suspected when the patient experiences frequent bouts of chest discomfort and pain either at rest or with minimal exertion for periods lasting up to 30 minutes.

Myocardial ischemia lasting more than 20 to 30 minutes may result in myocardial necrosis and infarction. Myocardial infarction produces prolonged pain that radiates to the left shoulder, arm, and jaw. In contrast to angina pectoris, the pain of myocardial infarction is unrelated to physical exertion and if untreated lasts for several hours. Myocardial infarction is occasionally painless.[5] Patients may also complain of dyspnea, palpitations, and diaphoresis. Diagnosis is made by serial electrocardiographic and enzyme studies.

Mitral valve prolapse may be associated with precordial or substernal chest pain of short or prolonged duration.[6] A late systolic murmur and mid-systolic click would suggest the disorder, and the echocardiogram may be useful in establishing the diagnosis. Patients with severe aortic stenosis or idiopathic hypertrophic subaortic stenosis may develop ischemic chest pain. Finally, coronary artery involvement in patients with Takayasu's disease, periarteritis nodosa, and progressive systemic sclerosis may also cause ischemic chest pain.

Pericardial. Sensory pain fibers originate in the parietal pericardium abutting the diaphragm. Pericardial pain is localized to the sternal and precordial areas, but may radiate to the epigastrium, neck, shoulders, and back. The pain is usually described as stabbing or knifelike and is aggravated by deep breathing, swallowing, turning, and twisting. Pain may decrease when the patient sits up and leans forward. Specific movements that increase the pain (such as turning over) may be helpful in distinguishing it from angina. Lateral diaphragmatic pericardial inflammation may produce epigastric and back pain similar to that experienced by patients with pancreatitis or cholecystitis.

Aortic. Patients with hypertension, Marfan's syndrome, aortic cystic medial necrosis, pregnancy, coarctation of the aorta, and chest trauma are at increased risk for aortic dissection.[7] The sudden onset of severe anterior chest pain or interscapular pain strongly suggests the diagnosis. The pain may resemble that of myocardial infarction but is often sharper and more likely to be referred to the interscapular areas and down the back, depending on the location and extent of the dissection. Proximal dissection and distal dissection are commonly associated with anterior chest pain and back pain, respectively. Proximal dissection may be associated with aortic regurgitation, pericardial tamponade, cerebrovascular accidents, or upper-extremity pulse deficits; distal dissection may cause pulse deficits in the lower extremities and spinal cord or renal ischemia or infarction. A widened mediastinum or aortic contour is found on chest x-ray film. Left-sided hemorrhagic pleural effusions caused by aortic bleeding may be present. Definitive diagnosis is confirmed by aortography.

Pulmonary. The pain associated with acute and chronic pulmonary hypertension is similar to that of angina pectoris and is produced by myocardial ischemia secondary to reduction in cardiac output and coronary blood flow.[8] Carcinoma of the lung with extension to the chest wall or brachial plexus may produce a boring, excrutiating, constant chest pain.

Gastrointestinal. Reflux esophagitis, abnormal motility, neoplasms, infections, or involvement of the esophagus with progressive systemic sclerosis may cause esophageal pain.[9-11] Midline esophageal pain radiates to the back, shoulders, and occasionally down the inner sides of the arms and closely resembles anginal pain. Perforated peptic ulcer, acute pancreatitis, gastric distention, and splenic flexure syndrome sometimes cause substernal pain that may be confused with ischemic cardiac pain.[11] Burning pain (heartburn) associated with dysphagia or regurgitation that worsens on assuming the recumbent position and improves with antacid therapy is characteristic of esophageal disorders. Upper gastrointestinal series, esophagrams, acid perfusion test (Bernstein test), esophagoscopy, and esophageal motility studies can aid in the proper diagnosis.[9]

Musculoskeletal. Local trauma or inflammation of the chest cage, muscles, bones, and cartilage are common causes of chest pain and localized tenderness. The pain usually begins after physical exercise, helping differentiate it from coronary pain, which occurs during exercise. As with pleuritic pain, deep inspiration may worsen chest wall pain. Muscular pain is reproduced by twisting movements of the chest, while pleuritic pain usually is not.

Chest pain of sudden or gradual onset, aggravated by coughing or deep breathing and localized to one or more upper cartilages, is found with Tietze's syndrome (costal chondritis). The affected cartilage is swollen and tender to palpation. Anterior chest pain can be caused by a herniated spinal disc with nerve root irritation, thoracic outlet syndromes, and herpes zoster.[12] Invasive malignancies or infections may cause persistent chest pain.

Functional. Acute anxiety can cause substernal or precordial pain or discomfort, palpitations, dyspnea, dizziness, and the feeling of impending death. The patient's disturbed emotional state and lack of objective evidence of organic heart disease are important clues distinguishing functional pain from pain of myocardial ischemia.

DaCosta's syndrome is a chronic anxiety state in which the patient complains of dyspnea, palpitations, fatigue, dizziness, and precordial or substernal sharp, stabbing chest pain. It usually occurs after exercise and lasts for many hours.[13] The pain-producing mechanisms are unknown.

CHEST PAIN IN SPECIFIC PULMONARY DISEASES

The following table lists characteristics of chest pain related to specific pulmonary diseases. A positive (+) sign signifies that chest pain is the chief complaint; a positive/negative (±) sign indicates that in a certain percent of patients chest pain may be the chief complaint; and a negative (−) sign means that chest pain may be present but is not the chief complaint. The severity of chest pain is classified as follows: 1 is mild—the patient is able to tolerate this chest pain without employing analgesics or narcotics; 2 is moderate—the chest pain is less tolerable and may require analgesics; and 3 is severe—the chest pain may be excrutiating, and narcotics are needed for relief.

Disease	Chief complaint of chest pain	Severity	Comments
Obstructive lung disease			
Uncommon			
6. Upper airway obstruction	−	1–2	Pain on swallowing is a common complaint of patients with chronic laryngeal infections (e.g., laryngeal tuberculosis).
Restrictive lung disease			
Common			
9. Pulmonary edema	±	1–3	Pulmonary edema *per se* does not cause chest pain, but if the pulmonary edema is secondary to an event such as acute myocardial infarction, pain is characteristic.
10. Thoracic cage deformities and abnormalities	−	1	Anterior chest pain is common in patients with ankylosing spondylitis, kyphoscoliosis, and thoracoplasty.

Disease	Chief complaint of chest pain	Severity	Comments
Uncommon			
16. Eosinophilic granuloma	−	1–2	Chest pain is unusual unless the patient suffers a pneumothorax, in which case stabbing anterior chest pain is common.
Pulmonary vascular disease			
Common			
17. Acute pulmonary embolism	−	2–3	The pain mimics the pain of acute myocardial infarction and is substernal. Pleuritic chest pain is common in patients with pulmonary infarction.
Uncommon			
18. Sickle cell disease	−	2–3	Pleuritic chest pain is common and is secondary to pleural effusions from either pulmonary infarction or pneumonia.
19. Recurrent pulmonary thromboembolism	−	1–2	Pleuritic chest pain is common, but chest pain mimicking angina pectoris has also been described.
20. Primary pulmonary hypertension	−	1–2	Exertional precordial pain occurs in up to 50% of these patients. Severe chest pain is rarely due to dissection of a main pulmonary artery.
Tumors of the lung, pleura, and mediastinum			
Common			
22. Carcinoma of the lung	±	1–3	Chest pain may be the chief complaint if the carcinoma spreads to the pleura, mediastinal structures, or chest wall. Patients with superior sulcus tumors experience intractable neck, chest, and arm pain even though the apical lesion may be small. Esophageal involvement leads to pain on swallowing.

Disease	Chief complaint of chest pain	Severity	Comments
23. Metastatic carcinoma of the lung	−	1–2	Pain is unusual unless the tumor involves pain-sensitive areas of the chest wall or pleura.

Infectious diseases of the lung

Common

Disease	Chief complaint of chest pain	Severity	Comments
26. Bacterial, mycoplasmal, and rickettsial pneumonias	±	1–3	Chest pain is secondary to parapneumonic effusions or empyemas and is usually pleuritic in nature.
27. Viral pneumonias	−	1–2	Pleuritic chest pain is uncommon but occasionally occurs in viral pneumonias.
28. Lung abscesses	−	1–3	Chest pain occurs with either pleural involvement or development of an empyema.
29. Tuberculosis	−	1–3	Pleuritic chest pain is common.

Uncommon

Disease	Chief complaint of chest pain	Severity	Comments
30. Atypical tuberculosis	−	1–2	
31. *Actinomyces* and *Nocardia*	±	1–3	Chest pain may be due to pleural involvement or direct invasion of the chest wall by actinomyces.
32. Mycoses	−	1–3	Pain is common and usually pleuritic in nature. Invasion of the chest wall can occur in certain of these infections, and constant pain may then be present.
35. Wegener's granulomatosis, its variants, and other vasculitides	−	1–2	Pleuritic chest pain has been described.

REFERENCES

1. Hyde L: Benign spontaneous pneumothorax. Ann Intern Med 56:746, 1962
2. Munsell WP: Pneumomediastinum. A report of 28 cases and review of the literature. JAMA 202:689, 1967

3. Silver MD, Baroldi G, Mariani F: The relationship between acute occlusive coronary thrombi and myocardial infarction studied in 100 consecutive patients. Circulation 61:219, 1980

4. Goldberg A, Reichek N, Wilson J et al: Nifedipine in the treatment of Prinzmetal's (variant) angina. Am J Cardiol 44:804, 1979

5. Cohn PF: Silent myocardial ischemia in patients with a defective anginal warning system. Am J Cardiol 45:697, 1980

6. Jeresaty RM: Mitral valve prolapse—Click syndrome. Prog Cardiovasc Dis 15:623, 1973

7. Slater EE, DeSanctis RW: Dissection of the aorta. Med Clin North Am 63:141, 1979

8. Sharma GV, Sasahara AA: Diagnosis and treatment of pulmonary embolism. Med Clin North Am 63:239, 1979

9. Pope CE: Esophageal function tests in the differential diagnosis of chest pain. In Chest Pain: Diagnostic Testing, pp 15–21. Philadelphia, Lea & Febiger, 1980

10. Vantrappen G, Janssens J, Hellemans J et al: Achalasia, diffuse esophageal spasm and related motility disorders. Gastroenterology 76:450, 1979

11. Winans CS: The role of endoscopy in the diagnosis of esophageal pain. In Chest Pain: Diagnostic Testing, pp 27–33. Philadelphia, Lea & Febiger, 1980

12. Davis D, Ritvo M: Osteoarthritis of the cervicodorsal spine (radiculitis) simulating coronary-artery disease. Clinical and roentgenologic findings. N Engl J Med 238:857, 1948

13. Wooley CF: Where are the diseases of yesteryear? DaCosta's syndrome, soldier's heart, the effort syndrome, neurocirculatory asthenia and the mitral valve prolapse syndrome. Circulation 53:749, 1976

5 · HEMOPTYSIS

ORHAN MUREN

DEFINITION

Hemoptysis is expectoration or coughing up of blood, bloody sputum, or blood-tinged sputum from the lungs or tracheobronchial tree. Hemoptysis may be confused with hematemesis, (vomiting of blood). Blood originating in the tracheobronchial tree is usually red, frothy, has an alkaline pH and contains hemosiderin-laden histiocytes. Respiratory symptoms, cough, a ticklish sensation in the throat, and blood produced by repeated coughing episodes strongly suggest the diagnosis of hemoptysis. Blood-stained sputum may be present for several days after an episode of hemoptysis.

In contrast, blood originating from the gastrointestinal tract is usually dark, often has a coffee-ground character, has an acid pH, and may contain food particles. The stools may be tarry and contain traces of blood following an episode of hematemesis. Many patients with hematemesis complain of dyspepsia.

MECHANISMS AND DIFFERENTIAL DIAGNOSIS

Expectorated blood may originate in the mouth, nose, pharynx, or larynx. These areas must be examined when the site of bleeding is unclear. Repeated expectoration of 2 ml to 3 ml or more of blood is associated with a serious underlying disease and outcome. In contrast, repeated streaky hemoptysis with vigorous coughing implies less serious disease and a better outcome. Streaky hemoptysis is usually due to chronic bronchitis, acute exacerbation of chronic bronchitis, or acute tracheobronchitis. Patients with bronchial carcinomas and bacterial pneumonias may also note streaky hemoptysis. Hemoptysis, especially a single episode of blood-streaked sputum, often remains unexplained even after complete investigation.

Massive hemoptysis is defined as coughing up 400 ml of blood within 3 hours or 600 ml of blood within 24 hours. The most common causes of massive hemoptysis are carcinoma of the lung, cavitary pulmonary disease secondary to quiescent necrotizing infections or tuberculosis, bronchiectasis, and active tuberculosis. The mortality rate is approximately 75%.[1,2] Surgery offers the best chance for survival in these patients.[3-5]

Hemoptysis may be caused by or associated with the following:

1. Intra-alveolar hemorrhage and diapedesis of red blood cells from the pulmonary microvasculature into the alveoli (acute pulmonary edema)
2. Necrosis of lung tissue with hemorrhage into the alveolar spaces (pulmonary infarction)
3. Rupture of distended endobronchial blood vessels (mitral stenosis)[6]
4. Ulceration and erosion of bronchial epithelium (bronchitis, broncholithiasis)
5. Sloughing of a caseous lesion into the tracheobronchial tree (tuberculosis)
6. Rupture of a pulmonary arteriovenous fistula (Osler–Weber–Rendu disease), bronchial artery–pulmonary venous collateral channels (bronchiectasis), and systemic blood vessel–pulmonary venous collateral channels (sequestration)[7-9]
7. Invasion of blood vessels (carcinoma of the lung)
8. Necrosis of lung tissue associated with inflammation and rupture of blood vessels (necrotizing pneumonias and some parasitic infections)[10-12]
9. Rupture of an aortic aneurysm into the tracheobronchial tree
10. Anticoagulants and immunosuppressive drugs causing intraparenchymal bleeding
11. Menses[13]
12. Malingering

HEMOPTYSIS IN SPECIFIC PULMONARY DISEASES

The following table lists characteristics of hemoptysis related to specific pulmonary diseases. A positive (+) sign signifies that hemoptysis is the chief complaint in a specific disease; a positive/negative (±) sign means that hemoptysis may be the chief complaint in a small percentage of patients; and a negative (−) sign means that hemoptysis may be present but is not the chief complaint. The severity of hemoptysis can be defined as follows: 0 is no hemoptysis; 1 is mild—occasionally blood-streaked sputum; 2 is moderate—persistent blood-streaked sputum and gross blood; 3 is severe—for example, massive bleeding.

Disease	Chief complaint of hemoptysis	Severity	Comments
Obstructive lung disease			
Common			
1. Chronic bronchitis	–	1–2	Fifty percent of all hemoptysis cases are due to chronic bronchitis. Although hemoptysis is usually due to superimposed acute respiratory infection, an underlying carcinoma as the cause of the bleeding must not be overlooked.
Uncommon			
4. Bronchiectasis	±	1–3	Oozing or rupture of bronchial artery–pulmonary artery communication results in hemoptysis. Hemoptysis may vary from blood-tinged sputum to expectoration of gross blood. Bronchiectasis accounts for 30% of all cases of gross hemoptysis.
5. Cystic fibrosis	–	1–2	Expectoration of blood-streaked sputum, especially during periods of acute respiratory infection, is relatively common.
6. Upper airway obstruction	–	1–2	Hemoptysis may be present when the upper airway obstruction is caused by necrotizing carcinomas or granulomas.
Restrictive lung disease			
Common			
8. Sarcoidosis	–	1–2	Hemoptysis is usually due to the presence of a fungus ball (e.g., aspergilloma) in a patient with advanced cystic sarcoidosis. Bleeding can be life threatening.

Disease	Chief complaint of hemoptysis	Severity	Comments
9. Pulmonary edema	–	1–2	Acute elevations of left atrial pressure, such as occur with myocardial infarction and mitral stenosis, can lead to diapedesis of red blood cells from the pulmonary vasculature into alveoli with the production of pinkish sputum. In addition, rupture of distended bronchial vessels may cause hemoptysis.
12. Inhalational or occupational lung diseases	–	1–2	The inhalational lung diseases that cause acute pulmonary edema (e.g., nitrogen dioxide exposure) can lead to hemorrhagic sputum production.

Uncommon

14. Goodpasture's syndrome	±	1–2	Massive hemoptysis is uncommon. Most patients experience episodes of minor hemoptysis.
15. Idiopathic pulmonary hemosiderosis	±	1–2	Minor hemoptysis is common and is often associated with sputum production. Massive hemoptysis is uncommon.

Pulmonary vascular diseases

Common

17. Acute pulmonary embolism	±	1–2	The sputum is usually blood streaked. It is uncommon for large quantities of blood to be expectorated. Hemoptysis can occur with pulmonary embolism alone and when the embolus is associated with pulmonary congestion or infarction.

Disease	Chief complaint of hemoptysis	Severity	Comments
Uncommon			
18. Sickle cell disease	−	1–2	Minor blood streaking may occur with either pulmonary infection or infarction. Gross hemoptysis is unusual.
Tumors of the lung, pleura, and mediastinum			
Common			
21. Carcinoma of the lung	±	1–3	Blood-streaked sputum or frankly bloody expectoration may be one of the earliest complaints from patients with carcinoma of the lung. Recurrent episodes of hemoptysis are characteristic of this condition. Severe hemoptysis may occur and can be terminal if the tumor is extensive.
23. Metastatic carcinoma of the lung	−	1–2	Hemoptysis is rare in this condition. Patients with metastatic bronchogenic carcinoma or osteogenic carcinoma (both are vascular tumors) may present with hemoptysis.
25. Bronchial adenoma	±	1–3	Recurrent episodes of hemoptysis are common, and hemoptysis can be massive.
Infectious disease of the lung			
Common			
26. Bacterial, mycoplasmal, and rickettsial pneumonias	−	1–2	Hemoptysis is common in necrotizing pneumonias due to staphylococci, klebsiella, and gram-negative organisms. It is uncommon in the usual bacterial, mycoplasmal, and rickettsial pneumonias. Persistent hemoptysis in patients with pneumonia should suggest an underlying carcinoma of the lung.

Disease	Chief complaint of hemoptysis	Severity	Comments
27. Viral pneumonias	–	1–2	Influenza or varicella pneumonias rarely cause hemoptysis.
28. Lung abscesses	–	1–2	Although blood streaking is common in patients with multiple small or single large lung abscesses, gross hemoptysis is distinctly uncommon. A patient may occasionally have gross hemoptysis that directly causes death.
29. Tuberculosis	±	1–3	Blood-streaked sputum is common. Hemoptysis may be the first manifestation of this disease. Massive hemoptysis may occasionally occur in patients with advanced cavitary tuberculosis.
Uncommon			
30. Atypical tuberculosis	–	1–2	
31. *Actinomyces* and *Nocardia*	–	1–2	
32. Mycoses	–	1–3	Hemoptysis is common in patients with a fungus ball or mycetoma. Hemoptysis in patients who are being treated with immunosuppressive agents can be due to a fungal infection.
Miscellaneous			
36. Wegener's granulomatosis, its variants, and other vasculitides	–	1–2	Hemoptysis may be present in patients with classical and limited Wegener's granulomatosis and necrotizing vasculitis.

REFERENCES

1. Crocco JA, Rooney JJ, Fankushen DS et al: Massive hemoptysis. Arch Intern Med 121:495, 1968

2. Editorial: Massive hemoptysis. Br Med J 3:669, 1969
3. Gottlieb LS, Hillberg R: Endobronchial tamponade therapy for intractable hemoptysis. Chest 67:482, 1975
4. Gourin A, Garzon AA: Control of hemorrhage in emergency pulmonary resection for massive hemoptysis. Chest 68:120, 1975
5. Mattox KL, Guinn GA: Emergency resection for massive hemoptysis. Ann Thorac Surg 17:377, 1974
6. Diamond MA, Genovese PD: Life threatening hemoptysis in mitral stenosis. Emergency mitral valve replacement resulting in rapid, sustained cessation of pulmonary bleeding. JAMA 215:441, 1971
7. Britt CI, Andrews NC, Klassen KP: Pulmonary arteriovenous fistula. Am J Surg 101:727, 1961
8. Rasmussen V: On haemoptysis, especially when fatal, in its anatomical and clinical aspects. Edinburgh Med J Part 1:385, 1868
9. Sade RM, Clouse M, Ellis FH, Jr: The spectrum of pulmonary sequestration. Ann Thorac Surg 18:644, 1974
10. Yang SP, Huang CT, Cheng CS et al: The clinical and roentgenological course of pulmonary paragonimiasis. Dis Chest 36:494, 1959
11. Murray HW: Pulmonary mucormycosis with massive fatal hemoptysis. Chest 68:65, 1975
12. Freundlich IM, Israel HL: Pulmonary aspergillosis. Clin Radiol 24:248, 1973
13. Rodman MH, Jones CW: Catamenial hemoptysis due to bronchial endometriosis. N Engl J Med 266:805, 1962

6 · WHEEZING

KEVIN R. COOPER

DEFINITION

A wheeze is an abnormally high-pitched sound produced by breathing through partially obstructed or narrowed airways.[1] Wheezing may be localized or diffusely audible, is more prominent during exhalation, and is associated with prolonged expiration. In contrast to wheezing, stridor is a continuous sound that is more prominent during inspiration and usually associated with upper airway obstruction.

MECHANISMS AND PATHOPHYSIOLOGY

The following factors may cause the airways to narrow.[2]

Bronchospasm. All airways from the trachea to the alveolar ducts are at least partially surrounded by a smooth-muscle cell layer that can contract circumferentially, leading to airway narrowing. Bronchospasm is a primary mechanism causing airway obstruction in patients with acute asthma and in some patients with chronic bronchitis.

Mucosal Edema. Airway mucosa thickening may be due to the infiltration of inflammatory cells and edema. This swelling encroaches on or completely obliterates the airway lumen. Mucosal edema is a major factor leading to airway obstruction in patients with chronic bronchitis and asthma.

Tortuosity of the Airways. The tracheobronchial tree undergoes symmetric dichotomous branching as it divides into smaller caliber airways. Necrotic or fibrotic processes adjacent to the airways or destruction of the airway-supporting structures (e.g., alveoli, cartilage) can cause constrictions, dilatations, and angulations of the tracheobronchial tree. This increased airway resistance may produce audible wheezing.

Loss of Elastic Support. During forced exhalation, intrathoracic pressure normally rises above the airway pressure, compressing the airways and increasing resistance to air flow. The greater the expiratory effort, the greater the dynamic compression (see Fig. 2–1). Airways larger than bronchioles contain some cartilage that helps resist this tendency to collapse, but bronchioles and alveolar ducts are supported primarily by their attachment to surrounding lung. These attachments are elastic so that airway support and airway diameter are greatest at high lung volumes and smallest at low lung volumes (Fig. 6–1).

A

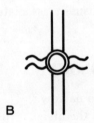

B

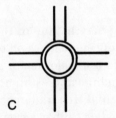

C

Fig. 6–1. The effects of different lung volumes on airway diameter. A, At low lung volumes near residual volume, the airway elastic supporting tissue is collapsed and airway size is small. B, At normal volumes near functional residual capacity, some of the elastic supporting structures have become turgid and the airway lumen enlarges. C, At large lung volumes near total lung capacity, all elastic tissue is stretched further, opening the airways.

At some point, the airway compressive forces overcome the supportive forces and air flow ceases. Airway closure occurs at relatively low lung volumes or below functional residual capacity in normal people, but in patients with destructive diseases of the elastic supporting structures (e.g., emphysema) airway closure occurs during relaxed tidal breathing. If virtually all airways are subject to dynamic compression during relaxed tidal breathing, exhalation will be prolonged and will require active effort (normal resting exhalation is passive and effortless).

Obstruction by Intraluminal Debris. Large amounts of material may accumulate within the airways. Like boulders in a shallow river, this material narrows the stream (airway) and changes air flow direction producing turbulence and eddy currents that increase resistance. These "boulders" are composed of mucus secretions, inflammatory cells, water, and (occasionally) aspirated foreign bodies.

Voluntary Contraction of the Airway Outlet. True wheezing can be simulated by voluntary apposition of the vocal cords during forced exhalation.[3] A patient may or may not be consciously aware of performing this voluntary maneuver. Wheezing may be generalized, and physical examination may not reveal its source. Laryngoscopy will confirm the diagnosis if voluntary contraction of the airway outlet is suspected.

CLINICAL CORRELATIONS

Cough and dyspnea are often found in patients who wheeze.[4] In fact, the symptom of wheezing is often not volunteered by the patient. Dyspnea produces a feeling of apprehension and distress and is common in patients with airway obstruction (see Chap. 1). Many of the factors that cause wheezing also stimulate receptors that initiate coughing.[5] Patients with asthma may present with cough as their only symptom and deny any history of wheezing (see Chap. 2).

Patients may be more distressed by the sensation of chest tightness than by the actual wheezing. The sensation of tightness may emanate from airway sensory receptors or from sensory signals in the chest wall that are triggered by air trapping and hyperinflation.

A decrease in wheezing means that either the airway obstruction is reversing or less air movement is taking place and airway obstruction is worsening. Wheezing first increases and then decreases during an increasingly severe asthmatic attack. A relatively silent chest in a patient with acute asthma is ominous.

HISTORICAL DATA

The physical examination is often normal or nonspecific at the time the patient seeks medical attention, so an accurate history is most important in the evaluation of wheezing. The following should be established:

1. The total duration of the symptom (e.g., when did it begin, at what age?)
2. The duration of individual wheezing attacks
3. The time of day when wheezing is most likely
4. The frequency of attacks
5. Specific precipitating factors such as smoke, odors, posture, specific exposures, air temperature and humidity, medication, and food[6,7]
6. Response to various forms of treatment, either self-administered or prescribed by physicians
7. The general progression of symptoms over time (e.g., whether they are becoming better or worse)[8]
8. The state of health and ventilatory ability between attacks (e.g., does the patient's breathing completely return to normal after resolution of the wheezing?)
9. Associated symptoms (e.g., dyspnea, cough, anxiety or depression, nasal stuffiness, postnasal drip, or facial flushing)
10. Any difficulties involving the upper airway (e.g., previous hoarseness or change in volume of the voice)
11. Evidence of congestive heart failure
12. Smoking history
13. Evidence of sinusitis

UNCOMMON CAUSES OF WHEEZING

A variety of rare pulmonary and nonpulmonary diseases are associated with wheezing: parasitic infections, particularly when associated with eosinophilia (the so-called PIE syndrome [pulmonary infiltration with eosinophilia]; an expanding aortic aneurysm that compresses a major airway; and intrabronchial endometriosis. It is possible for patients to wheeze on cue because wheezing can be voluntarily produced or deliberately exaggerated. Laryngoscopy during a wheezing episode will confirm that the vocal cords are the source of sound if the patient is malingering.

WHEEZING IN SPECIFIC PULMONARY DISEASES

The following table lists characteristics of wheezing related to specific pulmonary diseases. A positive (+) sign signifies wheezing is the chief complaint in a specific disease; a positive/negative (±) sign means that wheezing *may* be the chief complaint in a small percentage of patients; and a negative (−) sign means that the wheezing may be present but *is not* the chief complaint. The severity of wheezing may be classified as follows: 1 is mild—noted by patient but does not affect activity; 2 is moderate—noted by patient, audible, and limiting activity; and 3 is severe—clearly audible and routine activity is impossible.

Disease	Chief complaint of wheezing	Severity	Comments
Obstructive lung disease			
Common			
1. Emphysema	−	1–2	A prolonged expiratory phase with or without associated wheezing is characteristic of emphysema. The expiratory airway compression in this disease is due to loss of elastic support (so-called floppy airways). In contrast to patients with asthma and chronic bronchitis, wheezing in patients with emphysema is poorly responsive to bronchodilator therapy.
2. Chronic bronchitis	±	1–3	Wheezing is a common complaint in patients with acute or chronic bronchitis. In the latter patients, wheezing may be initially noted only during chest colds. Wheezing is more frequent or continuously present as the disease progresses.

Disease	Chief complaint of wheezing	Severity	Comments
3. Asthma	+	1–3	Asthma is the most common cause of wheezing in patients under 40 years of age. Wheezing responds dramatically to bronchodilator therapy, except during status asthmaticus. Intermittent wheezing is a cardinal feature of asthma because most patients are wheeze-free between asthmatic attacks.
Uncommon			
4. Bronchiectasis	±	1–3	Wheezing is intermittent but not as variable in intensity as in asthma patients. The wheezing may be either localized or diffuse depending on the extent of the bronchiectasis. Wheezing is due to retained secretions, distorted airway architecture, and mucosal edema.
5. Cystic fibrosis	±	1–3	Wheezing is similar to that in patients with bronchiectasis but begins at an earlier age.
6. Upper airway obstruction	±	1–3	Inspiratory wheezing (stridor) is a common complaint of patients with extrathoracic upper airway obstruction, but expiratory wheezing may also be present. Stridor occurs when airway narrowing is severe and associated with a 75% decrease in the cross-sectional diameter of the trachea. Stridor noted at rest is an ominous finding, indicating imminent danger of acute airway obstruction. Stridor noted during exercise or with increased minute ventilation implies a lesser degree of airway obstruction.
Restrictive lung disease			
Common			
7. Interstitial fibrosis	–	1	Wheezing is distinctly uncommon except during the later stages of this disease when parenchymal scarring may result in traction and deformation of the airways.

Disease	Chief complaint of wheezing	Severity	Comments
8. Sarcoidosis	−	1	Sarcoidosis is distinct from many other forms of interstitial lung disease because it has a propensity to involve airways. Twenty percent of patients have evidence of obstructive defect on spirometry, and a small percentage of this group may wheeze.
9. Pulmonary edema	−	1–3	Wheezing is very common in patients with congestive heart failure secondary to left ventricular dysfunction. This diagnosis should be suspected in every middle-aged or older person who complains of wheezing, particularly if the initial episode of wheezing occurs in an older individual. Wheezing may be the primary or only symptom of congestive heart failure.
10. Thoracic cage deformities and abnormalities	−	1	Mechanical distortion of the tracheobronchial tree can lead to localized or generalized wheezing in a small percentage of these patients.
12. Inhalational or occupational pulmonary diseases	±	1–3	Many occupational exposures may induce bronchospasm or lead to chronic bronchitis; wheezing is therefore a common complaint in these patients. Wheezing is uncommon in inhalational or occupational diseases that involve the interstitium.
Uncommon			
13. Hypersensitivity pneumonitis	−	1–3	Approximately one third of patients experience early onset of wheezing after inhaling the offending substances.
14. Eosinophilic granuloma	−	1	Airway compression due to the granulomatous process and interstitial fibrosis may produce traction and deformity of the airways, resulting in wheezing.

Disease	Chief complaint of wheezing	Severity	Comments
Pulmonary vascular disease			
Common			
17. Acute pulmonary embolism	–	1–2	Although up to 85% of patients with pulmonary embolism have bronchospasm by pulmonary function studies, only 10 to 15% of these patients have clinically evident wheezing. Wheezing is postulated to be due to bronchoconstriction secondary to the release of histamine, slow-reacting substances of anaphylaxis, and serotonin.
Uncommon			
19. Recurrent pulmonary thromboembolism	–	1–2	When accompanied by wheezing, recurrent pulmonary emboli may be mistaken for repeated attacks of asthma.
21. Pulmonary veno-occlusive disease	–	1–2	Wheezing may occur secondary to airway edema.
Tumors of the lung, pleura, and mediastinum			
Common			
22. Carcinoma of the lung	–	1–3	Wheezing, which is localized to one area of the chest, suggests discrete airway obstruction. Tumor involvement of the trachea or both mainstem bronchi results in generalized wheezing. Many patients with carcinoma of the lung wheeze because of the associated bronchitis and emphysema.
23. Metastatic carcinoma of the lung	–	1–2	Breast, kidney, gastrointestinal tract, and gonadal tumors may cause endobronchial metastases resulting in partial airway obstruction and wheezing. Gastrointestinal carcinoid tumors may cause wheezing when associated with carcinoid syndrome due to the release of serotonin and

Disease	Chief complaint of wheezing	Severity	Comments
			bradykinins. External impingment of metastatic tumor on a large airway can also result in wheezing.
Uncommon			
25. Bronchial adenoma	+	2–3	Wheezing is a common complaint. A unilateral wheeze in a relatively young person should alert the physician to the possibility of a bronchial adenoma. A previously incorrect diagnosis of bronchial asthma is common in patients who are eventually proven to have these tumors.
Infectious diseases of the lung			
Common			
26. Bacterial, mycoplasmal, and rickettsial pneumonias	–	1–2	Partial airway occlusion from edema and sputum accumulation can cause wheezing in patients with bacterial pneumonias.
28. Lung abscesses	–	1–2	Patients with solitary lung abscesses and persistent wheezing should be evaluated for foreign body aspiration or an underlying partially obstructing endobronchial carcinoma.
29. Tuberculosis	–	1–2	Wheezing can be caused by compression secondary to large lymph nodes or airway distortion due to fibrosis. Tuberculosis only rarely involves the larynx directly, causing stridor, expiratory wheezing, or both.
Miscellaneous			
34. Aspiration lung disease	–	1–3	Airway edema and bronchospasm commonly occur following inhalation of gastric juices. Persistent localized wheezing suggests the possibility of foreign body aspiration.

Disease	Chief complaint of wheezing	Sever-ity	Comments
36. Wegener's granulomatosis, its variants, and other vasculitides	−	1–2	Wheezing in patients with Wegener's granulomatosis may occur if the granulomatous process causes major airway compression. In patients with bronchocentric granulomatosis, a rare variant of Wegener's granulomatosis, the granulomatous process involves the bronchi. Some of these patients have bronchial asthma, whereas others exhibit wheezing secondary to bronchial obstruction. Patients with Churg–Strauss vasculitides have eosinophilia and wheezing.

REFERENCES

1. Forgacs P: Lung Sounds. London, Baillière Tindall, 1978
2. West JB: Respiratory Physiology—The Essentials, 2nd ed. Baltimore, Williams & Wilkins, 1979
3. Cormier YF, Camus P, Desmeules MJ: Non-organic acute upper airway obstruction. Description and diagnostic approach. Am Rev Respir Dis 121:147, 1980
4. DeGowin EL, DeGowan RL: Bedside Diagnostic Examination, 2nd ed. New York, Macmillan, 1971
5. Corrao WM, Braman SS, Irwin RS: Chronic cough as the sole presenting manifestation of bronchial asthma. N Engl J Med 300:633, 1979
6. Ramsdell JW: Aspergillus lung disease. In Bardow RA, Stool EW, Moser KM (ed): Manual of Clinical Problems in Pulmonary Medicine, pp 170–175. Boston, MA, Little, Brown, & Co, 1980
7. Seaton A: Occupational asthma. In Morgan WKC, Seaton A (eds): Occupational Lung Diseases, pp 115–123. Philadelphia, W B Saunders, 1975
8. Traver GA, Cline MG, Burrows B: Predictors of mortality in chronic obstructive disease: A 15-year followup study. Am Rev Respir Dis 119:895–902, 1979

7 · ALTERED MENTAL STATUS, HEADACHE, AND COMA

THEODORE FEINSON

DEFINITION

Several interrelated factors determine an individual's mental status including sufficient quantities of oxygen in the cerebral blood, maintenance of normal cerebral spinal fluid acid–base relationships and electrolyte concentration, and maintenance and integrity of the cranium and its contents.[1] Changes in mental status occur along a continuum ranging from subtle alterations in cognition to coma.

MECHANISMS

General

Cerebrospinal fluid (CSF) hydrogen ion (H$^+$) concentration is the most important determinent of the level of consciousness.[2] Small decreases in oxygen tension have little effect on brain metabolism, but increases in carbon dioxide tension presumably decrease central nervous system function by increasing glucose use. Carbon dioxide is freely and rapidly diffusable across the blood brain barrier.[3] Serum bicarbonate is the major extracellular buffer; it diffuses poorly and is actively transported slowly into the CSF. The CSF Pco_2 climbs rapidly while the bicarbonate increases slowly, leading to local acidosis in patients with acute hypercapnea. The patient's mental status will deteriorate during this acute phase.[4] The CSF pH normalizes as HCO$_3$ concentration increases in chronic compensated respiratory acidosis. An altered mental status is less common in patients with chronic hypercapnea. In patients with respiratory alkalosis, metabolic acidosis, or alkalosis, the CSF pH deviates less from baseline values, and mental status changes are not as severe as in patients with acute hypercapnea.

Specific

Altered mental status in patients with pulmonary disease is ultimately due to cerebral cellular dysfunction from one of the following causes: cerebral hypoxia, direct brain involvement by the disease process, and electrolyte imbalances.

Cerebral hypoxia can be caused by cerebral arterial hypoxemia (decreased oxygen carrying capacity of the arterial blood) and decreased cerebral blood flow. Cerebral arterial hypoxemia occurs when the oxygen concentration (FIO_2) of the inspired air is low, as at high altitudes; when there is $\dot{V}/\dot{Q}$ mismatching, with intrapulmonic or intracardiac shunting; with abnormal diffusion of oxygen from the alveoli to the pulmonary capillaries; or when hypoventilation is present. $\dot{V}/\dot{Q}$ mismatch is the most common cause of hypoxemia in a wide variety of lung diseases.

Anemia and carbon monoxide inhalation reduce the oxygen carrying capacity of the blood. Hemolysis-induced anemia occurs in mycoplasma infection, systemic lupus erythematosis, lymphoma, and bacterial pneumonia. Various medications such as penicillin are used in the therapy of lung diseases and can cause hemolysis.

Cerebral blood flow may be reduced as a result of primary cardiac or pulmonary dysfunction, and hypoxemia itself may reduce cardiac function and induce arrhythmias. Massive pulmonary embolism can decrease right ventricular outflow; the myocardium and pericardium may be invaded by metastatic lung cancer, sarcoidosis, or infection; and pericardial healing after infection (e.g., tuberculosis) may lead to pericardial fibrosis and constriction. When cerebral blood flow decreases and cellular hypoxia ensues, lactic acidosis from anaerobic metabolism further alters cerebral function.

Sarcoid granulomas, brain abscesses secondary to pneumonia, tuberculosis, and metastatic carcinoma can *directly involve the brain* by forming intracranial masses. The patient's mental status is altered through displacement of brain tissue, compression of blood vessels, and seizure activity.[5] Focal neurologic deficits usually accompany this altered mental status.

Encephalitis and meningitis are common in viral, rickettsial, and *Legionella* infections. Simultaneous pulmonary and meningeal involvement occur in connective tissue disease such as systemic lupus erythematosis.

Electrolyte imbalances can also alter cerebral function. Hyponatremia secondary to inappropriate secretion of antidiuretic hormone (IADH) is common in patients with bronchogenic carcinoma, bacterial pneumonia and tuberculosis. Hypercalcemia from bony extension of a carcinoma or through elaboration of humoral substances such as parathyroidlike substance and prostaglandins can cause confusion and coma.

SYMPTOMS

As $Paco_2$ increases, cerebral arterial vessels dilate causing vascular headaches characterized by generalized throbbing and pulsatile pain over the entire cranium.[6] Hypercapnea worsens during sleep in patients with lung disease, and early morning headaches are often the first manifestation of hypercapnea. Headaches may be present throughout the day as the hypercapnea becomes persistent.

Headaches may also be due to intracerebral masses. In contrast to the headache associated with hypercapnea, headaches associated with a cerebral mass are usually localized to the site of the lesion and are continuous and nonpulsatile.[6]

Regardless of the specific cause, the stages but not the rate of mental deterioration are approximately the same in individual patients. Cognitive defects are first noted, followed by flattened affect. Memory, insight, and thought processes deteriorate and the mind wanders. The patient is easily distracted and conversation may resemble stream-of-consciousness thought. Headaches, tremors, asterixis, and myoclonus are common associated findings, and patients usually perceive these latter uncontrollable movements as nervousness.[5]

Both visual and auditory hallucinations are possible, and nightmares are. common in patients with hypercapnea. Finally, alertness is affected: agitation, progressive drowsiness, and disorientation may precede the development of stupor and coma.

ALTERED MENTAL STATUS, HEADACHE, AND COMA IN SPECIFIC PULMONARY DISEASES

The following table lists the proposed mechanisms responsible for the altered mental status, headache, or coma in patients with specific pulmonary diseases. Special characteristics of altered mental status, headache, or coma in specific diseases are discussed under Comments.

Disease	Mechanisms responsible for altered mental status, headache, or coma	Comments
Obstructive lung disease		
Common		
2. Chronic bronchitis	Hypercapnea, hypoxemia	Morning frontal headaches are common. Altered mental status and coma are common with acute exacerbation and worsening of the arterial blood gases.
3. Asthma	Hypercapnea, hypoxemia	Altered mental status and coma are associated with severe airway obstruction and are poor prognostic signs.
Uncommon		
6. Upper airway obstruction	Hypercapnea, hypoxemia	Coma and altered mental status are found with acute and total obstruction.
Restrictive lung disease		
Common		
8. Sarcoidosis	Central nervous system lesions, hypercapnea, electrolyte abnormalities	Altered mental status is uncommon, but may be due to sarcoidal involvement of the central nervous system.
9. Neuromuscular disorders	Hypercapnea, hypoxemia	
10. Inhalational or occupational pulmonary diseases	Electrolyte abnormalities	Certain inhaled substances may directly affect the central nervous system.
Pulmonary vascular diseases		
Common		
17. Acute pulmonary embolism	Hypoxemia, decreased cardiac output	Altered mental status is much more common than coma or headache.

Disease	Mechanisms responsible for altered mental status, headache, or coma	Comments
Tumors of the lung, pleura, and mediastinum		
Common		
22. Carcinoma of the lung	Central nervous system metastasis, decreased cerebral blood flow, and electrolyte abnormalities	Headaches are often caused by metastatic lesions to the brain. Altered mental status can be due to hyponatremia or hypercalcemia.
23. Metastatic carcinoma of the lung	Central nervous system mass lesions, electrolyte abnormalities	
Infectious diseases of the lung		
Common		
26. Bacterial, mycoplasmal, and rickettsial pneumonias	Hypoxemia, decreased cardiac output, central nervous system involvement	Altered mental status is common in these diseases and may be related to associated meningitis, vasculitis, or fevers.
27. Viral pneumonias	Central nervous system involvement, meningitis	Meningismus is common and may cause headaches and altered mental status.
29. Tuberculosis	Central nervous system involvement, decreased cardiac output	Meningitis may cause altered mental status, coma, and headache. The decreased cardiac output may be due to tuberculous pericardial involvement with constrictive pericarditis.
Uncommon		
31. *Actinomyces* and *Nocardia*	Central nervous system involvement	Brain abscesses are common with *Nocardia* infections.
32. Mycoses	Central nervous system involvement	Brain abscesses and meningitis are common with cryptococcal infections.
33. Sleep apnea and central hypoventilation syndromes	Hypercapnea, hypoxemia	Headache, altered mental status, and personality changes are common.

REFERENCES

1. Posner JB, Swanson AG, Plum F: Acid–base balance in cerebrospinal fluid. Arch Neurol 12:479–496, 1965
2. Posner JB, Plum F: Spinal-fluid pH and neurologic symptoms in systemic acidosis. N Engl J Med 277:605–613, 1967
3. Miller AL, Hawkins RA, Veech RL: Inhibition of brain glucose utilization by CO_2. J Neurosurg 25:553–558, 1975
4. Sieker HO, Hickam JB: Carbon dioxide intoxication. Medicine 35:389–423, 1956
5. Plum F, Posner JB (eds): Diffuse and metabolic brain diseases causing stupor and coma. In The Diagnosis of Stupor and Coma, pp 142–216. Philadelphia, FA Davis, 1980
6. Ryan RE, Sr, Ryan RE, Jr: Headache and Head Pain: Diagnosis and Treatment, pp 321–322. St. Louis, MO, CV Mosby, 1978

8 · ANOREXIA AND WEIGHT LOSS

FREDERICK L. GLAUSER

DEFINITION

Anorexia is defined as diminished appetite associated with aversion to food. Weight loss, a decrease in body weight of greater than 10% from baseline values, is the consequence of prolonged anorexia.

MECHANISMS

Anorexia and weight loss in patients with gastrointestinal disorders are commonly caused by nausea, vomiting, diarrhea, intestinal obstruction, or malabsorption. The mechanisms responsible for anorexia and weight loss in patients with certain forms of pulmonary and cardiac disease and in those with active neoplastic processes (e.g., carcinoma) are poorly understood, but it is accepted that they are not attributable to intestinal obstruction, sepsis, endocrine disorders, or other anatomic lesions.[1]

Dietary factors. Patients with cancer, advanced obstructive or restrictive lung disease, and cardiac disorders suffer from anorexia, and the etiology is poorly understood.[2-7] Many cancer patients ascribe their diminished appetite to an alteration in taste.[8,9] Increased intracranial pressure from metastatic tumors can cause pernicious vomiting.

Patients with chronic obstructive pulmonary disease (COPD) complain of early satiety after ingesting small quantities of food. This satiety may be due to gastric dilatation with subsequent impingement of the stomach on the diaphragm. This is associated with hypoxemia or increased carbon dioxide production from carbohydrate metabolism. Patients with COPD may also experience gastric irritation and ulceration.

Medicines. Digitalis preparations, aminophylline, beta-adrenergic agonists (terbutaline, metaproterenol), and steroids cause gastric irritation and anorexia with subsequent weight loss.

Hypermetabolism. The increased work of breathing in patients with limited cardiac and pulmonary reserves elevates their caloric needs, but the inability to increase food intake causes weight loss. An increase in sympathetic nervous discharge leading to elevated catecholamine levels has been reported in patients with both cor pulmonale and severe left ventricular failure. The catabolic action of this excess catecholamine leads to tissue breakdown and weight loss. Elevated endogenous steroid levels from adrenocorticotropic hormone (ACTH)-producing lung tumors causes weight loss secondary to the known catabolic effect of this hormone.

Cellular hypoxia. Tissue catabolism results from tissue oxygen delivery inadequate for metabolic demands. Severe arterial hypoxemia and decreased cardiac output are found in many patients with chronic lung disease; consequently, a decreased supply of nutrients and oxygen to the peripheral musculature and organs leads to weight loss. Although arterial hypoxemia is not a problem in patients with cardiac cachexia, the low cardiac output limits peripheral tissue oxygen and nutritional delivery.

Abnormal external losses. Vasoactive intestinal peptide (VIP)-producing tumors cause diarrhea.[10] As mentioned, various drugs including antimetabolites and alkylating agents can cause nausea, vomiting, and diarrhea.

Iatrogenic factors. The most common iatrogenic causes of anorexia and weight loss are associated with specific drugs. Cancer treatment itself predisposes to nutritional problems. Esophagitis and strictures may follow lower neck and mediastinal radiation.[11] Corticosteroid administration can cause fluid and electrolyte problems, nitrogen and calcium losses, and hyperglycemia. Surgery increases metabolic demands at the same time the patient's oral intake decreases.

ANOREXIA AND WEIGHT LOSS IN SPECIFIC PULMONARY DISEASES

The following table lists certain characteristics of anorexia and weight loss in relation to specific pulmonary diseases. The presence and severity of the anorexia can be classified as follows: 0 means anorexia not present, and appetite is normal; 1 is mild—food intake decreases by about 25%; 2 is moderate—food intake decreases by 25% to 50%; 3 is severe—food intake decreases by more than 50%. Weight loss can be classified as follows: 0 means weight loss not present; 1 is mild (about 10%); 2 is moderate (10% to 15%); 3 is severe (more than 15%). If anorexia or weight loss is the chief complaint of a specific disease process, it is noted under Comments.

Disease	Presence and severity		Comments
	Ano-rexia	Weight loss	
Obstructive lung disease			
Common			
1. Emphysema	1–3	1–3	Anorexia and weight loss are common complaints in patients with advanced emphysema. The diaphragm is affected by this generalized muscle wasting; this leads to easy fatigability and worsening respiratory failure. Many patients suffer acute weight loss after respiratory infection and never return to baseline weights.
2. Chronic bronchitis	0–1	1–2	Patients with cor pulmonale and peripheral edema, anasarca, and ascites are difficult to evaluate with regard to weight loss but it is commonly found that their dry weights are less than their ideal weights following diuresis. Anorexia and weight loss are not as great a problem in these patients as in those with emphysema.

Disease	Presence and severity		Comments
	Ano-rexia	Weight loss	
Uncommon			
4. Bronchiectasis	1–2	1–2	Weight loss is common in patients with diffuse bronchiectasis. It is related to the increased work of breathing and the effects of recurrent and persistent infections.
5. Cystic fibrosis	1–3	2–3	Weight loss is due to the increased work of breathing, recurrent and persistent infections, and pancreatic insufficiency with malabsorption.
6. Upper airway obstruction	0–1	1–2	Infectious laryngitis and carcinoma of the trachea are associated with anorexia and weight loss.
Restrictive lung disease			
Common			
7. Interstitial fibrosis	0–2	0–2	Patients with advanced disease associated with respiratory failure complain of anorexia and weight loss.
9. Pulmonary edema	0–1	0–2	Patients suffering from cardiomyopathies or severe coronary artery disease that limit cardiac output experience weight loss (cardiac cachexia)[12]
10. Thoracic cage deformities	0–1	1–2	Weight loss is common in patients with deforming kyphoscoliosis, extensive fibrothorax, and thoracoplasties.
11. Neuromuscular disorders	0–1	1–2	Patients with chronic poliomyelitis, muscular dystrophy, or multiple sclerosis have muscle wasting.
12. Inhalational or occupational pulmonary diseases	0–1	0–1	Weight loss is not encountered in acute inhalational lung disease, although transient anorexia may be present. Respiratory failure with weight loss occurs in patients with advanced disease from silicosis and asbestosis.

Disease	Presence and severity		Comments
	Ano-rexia	Weight loss	
Uncommon			
14. Goodpasture's syndrome	1–2	1–2	Anorexia and weight loss are common as with any other acute, serious disease.
15. Idiopathic pulmonary hemosiderosis	1–2	1–2	
Pulmonary vascular disease			
Uncommon			
18. Sickle cell disease	1–2	1–3	Fever, recurrent pneumonias, and increased work of breathing all contribute to the weight loss in this chronic disease.
Tumors of the lung, pleura, and mediastinum			
Common			
22. Carcinoma of the lung	1–3	2–3	Weight loss of 15 pounds or more is a poor prognostic sign and suggests distant metastasis. Anorexia may be a presenting and chief complaint in these patients.
23. Metastatic carcinoma of the lung	1–3	1–3	Weight loss may be the chief complaint.
Uncommon			
24. Malignant mesothelioma	2–3	2–3	Weight loss may be profound.
Infectious diseases of the lung			
Common			
26. Bacterial, mycoplasmal, rickettsial pneumonias	1–3	1–2	Weight loss is secondary to anorexia, decreased oral intake, fever, and infection. Rocky Mountain spotted fever can run a prolonged course and be associated with significant weight loss.
28. Lung abscesses	1–3	2–3	Anorexia, nausea, vomiting, and fever all contribute to weight loss.

Disease	Presence and severity		Comments
	Ano-rexia	Weight loss	
29. Tuberculosis	1–3	2–3	Anorexia and weight loss are common in patients with cavitary tuberculosis or tuberculous pneumonia. Many patients are initially misdiagnosed as having carcinoma of the lung because of the extreme muscle wasting.
Uncommon			
30. Atypical tuberculosis	1–2	2–3	This chronic debilitating disease is commonly associated with weight loss.
31. *Actinomyces* and *Nocardia*	1–2	2–3	
32. Mycoses	1–2	2–3	
Miscellaneous			
35. Pulmonary alveolar proteinosis	1–2	1–2	
36. Wegener's granulomatosis, its variants, and other vasculitides	1–2	2–3	

REFERENCES

1. Shils NE: Nutritional problems induced by cancer. Med Clin North Am 63:109, 1979
2. Young VR: Energy metabolism and requirements in cancer patients. Cancer Res 37:2336, 1977
3. Shils NE: Nutrition and neoplasia. In Goodhart R, Shils M (eds): Modern Nutrition in Health and Disease, 6th ed. Philadelphia, Lee & Febiger, 1979
4. DeWys W: Working conference on the anorexia and cachexia of neoplastic disease. Cancer Res 30:2816, 1976
5. Morrison SD: Origins of anorexia and neoplastic disease. Am J Clin Nutr 31:1014, 1978

6. Lertzman MM, Cherniack RH: Rehabilitation of patients with chronic obstructive pulmonary disease. Am Rev Respir Dis 114:1145, 1976
7. Hunter AM, Carey MA, Larsh HW: Nutritional status of patients with chronic obstructive pulmonary diseases. Am Rev Respir Dis 124:376–381, 1981
8. DeWys WD, Walter K: Abnormalities and taste sensation in cancer patients. Cancer 36:1888, 1975
9. Williams LR, Cohen MH: Altered taste threshold in lung cancer. Am J Clin Nutr 31:122, 1978
10. Pearse AGE, Polak JM, Bloom SR: The newer gut hormones: Cellular sources, physiology, pathology, and clinical aspects. Gastroenterology 72:746, 1977
11. Klipstein FA, Smarth G: Intestinal structure and function in neoplastic disease. Am J Dig Dis 14:887, 1969
12. Buchanan N, Cane RD, Kinsley R et al: Gastrointestinal absorption studies in cardiac cachexia. Intensive Care Med 3:89, 1977

9 · FEVER, CHILLS, AND NIGHTSWEATS

R. PAUL FAIRMAN

DEFINITION

Fever is a disease-induced elevation of body temperature to higher than 100.5°F or 38°C measured orally or higher than 101.5°F or 38.5°C measured rectally. Normal body temperature is maintained in a narrow range by central nervous system control, and fever is an elevation in the set point of this central nervous system thermostat. A balance between heat production and heat loss is maintained at any new thermal set point. The normal diurnal pattern is usually still observed in an exaggerated form.[1-4]

A chill is the subjective perception of inward trembling or cold that usually precedes a rapid rise in body temperature. It is often accompanied by generalized involuntary muscle tremors.[5] Nightsweats are abnormally increased nocturnal sweating that accompanies a nocturnal decline in body temperature.

MECHANISMS

Normal Body Temperature

Normal body temperature varies depending on where it is measured. The normal range for an oral temperature is between 97°F (36.1°C) and 99.6°F

(37.6°C). Oral temperatures may be significantly altered by ingestion of hot or cold liquids.

The normal rectal temperature is approximately 0.7°F (0.4°C) higher than the oral temperature, with axillary temperatures a similar amount lower. Rectal temperature determinations are preferable in patients who cannot keep their mouth closed during the measurement. Nevertheless, the traditional respect for rectal temperature measurements is misplaced. In contrast to rectal temperatures, oral and axillary temperature measurements show rapid and parallel responses to changes in body heat content. There is therefore no rational basis for the idea that rectal temperatures are somehow intrinsically more representative than oral temperatures.

Temperature in other portions of the body varies considerably. For example, the skin of the hands and feet is 5°F (2.7°C) to 20°F (11.1°C) below that of the oral cavity and the liver is warmer than blood. The hottest temperatures are recorded in exercising muscle, which reach highs of 107°F (41.7°C).

Diurnal variation in body temperature is normal with the maximal reading usually reached between 8 PM and 11 PM and the lowest between 4 AM and 6 AM (Fig. 9–1). Despite changes in environmental temperature, diet, or physical activity, this 2- to 3-degree variation is constant. The pattern of variation may be inverted in persons accustomed to nocturnal employment; however, some people adapt more readily to a new cycle whereas others retain the old cycle for many weeks.[1,2]

Regulation of Body Temperature

Body temperature is normally maintained within a narrow range by a delicate balance between heat production and heat loss. The set point of the hypothalmic thermoregulatory system is maintained through physiologic and behavioral mechanisms. Sweating and cutaneous vessel vasodilatation increase heat loss when it is hot, while vasoconstriction and shivering conserve heat or produce more heat when it is cold. The central nervous system integrates the processes that balance heat loss and heat production. A slight change in one must be compensated for by a change in the other.

Sources of Body Heat

Small quantities of heat are derived from the sun, heating fixtures, or other external sources. The internal combustion of food contributes up to one half of the normal heat production at rest. Brain and muscle metabolism contribute to most of the remainder. Muscles can produce as much as 90% of total body heat during strenuous labor.

Heat Elimination

Conduction of heat to cooler objects and warming ingested food minimally reduce body heat. Most heat is lost through radiation, evaporation, and

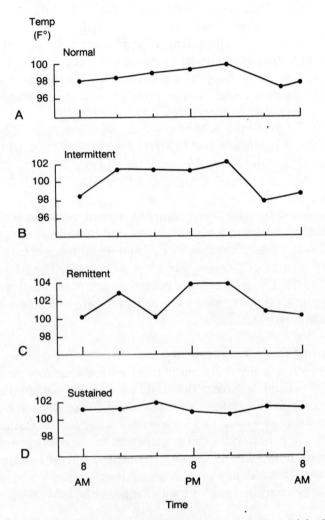

Fig. 9-1. Classic temperature patterns. *A,* Normal body temperature—the highest temperature occurs in the evening. *B,* Intermittent temperature—the temperature remains elevated throughout most of the day, but at some point (e.g., 4 AM in this example) the temperature returns to normal. *C,* remittent fever—the temperature waxes and wanes, never returning to normal. *D,* Sustained temperature—the temperature remains elevated without marked fluctuations.

convection. Radiation is the transfer of heat from a warmer object to a cooler one by electromagnetic waves. It accounts for approximately 60% of body heat elimination. At rest, even when sweating is not apparent, approximately one fourth to one fifth of total body heat is lost by evaporation through conversion of liquid to vapor. Sweating greatly increases this proportion. The remainder of body heat is lost to circulating air by convection.

Regulation of Temperature by the Central Nervous System

Body temperature regulation depends on an intact hypothalamus. Removal of this organ in animals causes unstable body temperature that parallels changes in environmental temperature. The exact manner by which the hypothalamus regulates temperature within narrow limits is unknown. There may be two anatomically distinct centers in the hypothalamus: one center may initiate sweating and vasodilatation (heat loss) while the other controls vasoconstriction and shivering (heat conservation). Activity in one area generally inhibits activity in the other. These hypothalamic responses are modified by peripheral stimuli arising from receptors in a number of sites, especially the skin and respiratory tract. The combined stimuli from all these receptors contribute to the temperature regulated by the hypothalamus.[3-5]

Fever is associated with elevation of the hypothalamic set point. The body maintains temperature within a narrow range through the usual control mechanisms despite increased temperature. Patients with sustained temperature elevations shiver when placed in a cool bath and sweat in a warm bath.

A reasonable explanation for the genesis of fever deals with two facts: fever is found in many kinds of disease processes, not only those infectious in nature; and fever results from diseases in practically any tissue of the body.

Bacterial pyrogens, also known as endotoxins, are complex lipopolysaccharides that form part of the bacterial cell wall in many bacteria and are responsible for fever in many infectious illnesses. Fever is common and is probably caused by the release of pyrogenic material from human phagocytic cells (Fig. 9–2) in certain noninfectious illnesses.[6-9] Either directly or through the release of prostaglandins, these pyrogens induce fever by altering the firing rate of neurons in the temperature sensitive region of the hypothalamus.

DIFFERENTIAL DIAGNOSIS

Clinical Fever, Chills, Sweating

Fever is one of the most ancient and widely recognized hallmarks of disease. The warm sensation of an established fever is well appreciated by

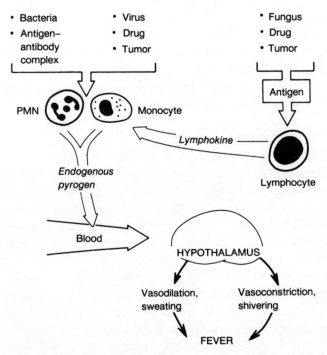

Fig. 9–2. Genesis of fever. A multitude of infectious and noninfectious stimuli interact with the neutrophil, and the monocytes release endogenous pyrogen into the blood stream. In addition, fungi, drugs, and tumor cells, through antigenic interaction, cause lymphocytes to release lymphokines that act on the neutrophils (PMNs) and monocytes to release endogenous pyrogens. Pyrogens circulate to the hypothalamus where vasoconstriction and vasodilation, sweating, and shivering are controlled.

most people. Constitutional symptoms include a general feeling of tiredness, anorexia, malaise, headache, restlessness, insomnia, and irritability. The pulse rate usually increases by 10 beats per minute for each degree (fahrenheit) above normal, and there is a slight increase in respiratory rate. The mouth is dry and the tongue coated.

Heat loss is minimized by peripheral vasoconstriction when the thermoregulatory system set point changes. The subjective consequence of this vasoconstriction is interpreted as chilliness, which may be mild and go unnoticed or may cause the patient to add another layer of clothing. The patient may shiver if increased heat production accompanies the febrile response. A severe attack of shivering is termed *rigor*. The patient who shivers uncontrollably and complains of feeling cold has a temperature that is rising sharply, usually as a result of rapid and widespread invasion of the host by bacteria or other infectious agents. The abrupt onset of fever with a chill is characteristic of certain diseases, such as pneumococcal pneumonia. Multiple chills frequently result from parasitic infections or localized abscesses. Chills can be associated with malignant diseases such as lymphoma and hypernephroma.

The usual diurnal variation persists because temperature regulation is normal in the febrile state, but at a higher set point. The temperature change is considerably greater than the 2- to 3-degree normal variation. Sweating (cooling) may be profuse when temperatures abruptly decline from their zenith to their nadir.

Normal humans increase sweat production within 30 minutes of falling asleep. This time corresponds to the normal nocturnal fall in temperature. Nocturnal sweating increases about threefold and is usually unnoticed because the temperature change is small. Sweating may increase threefold to fivefold in febrile patients. The patient experiences nightsweats when sweating increases eightfold. Nightsweats assumes clinical importance when the bed clothes or pillow cases become soaked. Any febrile disorder can be associated with nightsweats, but it is commonly experienced in patients with tuberculosis, Hodgkin's disease, lung abscesses, bacterial endocarditis, and so on.

Fever Patterns

Specific fever patterns have been recognized for decades. It has been suggested that patterns have special diagnostic significance with respect to infections by specific microorganisms, but this belief is not substantiated and usually cannot be applied to individual patients. Nevertheless, because this concept is widely taught, three patterns are worth describing (Fig. 9–1). In *intermittent fever*, the temperature is variably elevated but returns to normal at some time during the day. If the temperature swings are extreme, this pattern is termed *hectic*. In *remittent fever*, the body temperature waxes and wanes by 2 or 3 degrees never returning to normal. Most infection related fevers are of this type. *Sustained (continuous) fever* demonstrates relatively little variation (less than 2 degrees) throughout the day and night.

SUMMARY

The following general rules may be applied to body temperature:

A temperature greater than 106°F (41.1°C) is usually not the result of an infectious process.

In both the very young and very old, the febrile response to a specific infection may be disproportionate to the severity of the infection.

Some serious disorders may be characterized by remarkably little fever, and conversely, trivial infections may cause temperature elevations of 104°F (40°C) to 105°F (40.6°C).

In an adult, a body temperature greater than 104°F (40°C) often indicates the presence of a bacterial pneumonia or pyelonephritis.

Intermittent fevers are often associated with nightsweats.

Drug fevers are usually sustained, and the body temperature may be considerably higher than the patient's clinical well-being suggests.

FEVER, CHILLS, AND NIGHTSWEATS IN SPECIFIC PULMONARY DISEASES

The following table lists whether fevers, chills, and nightsweats are specific complaints in certain pulmonary diseases. A zero (0) indicates that fever, chills, and nightsweats do not occur; 1 is mild—fever lower than 101.5°F (38.6°C) orally, one or two chills, and nightsweats that does not soak the bed; 2 is moderate—fever of 101.5°F (38.6°C) to 103.5°F (39.7°C), repeated chills, and nightsweats that soaks the bed; 3 is fever higher than 103.5°F (39.7°C), repeated shaking chills or rigors, and nightsweats requiring a change of clothes and bed sheets. Specific comments, including whether fever, chills, or nightsweats are the chief complaint of any specific disease, are also included.

Disease	Specific complaint	Severity	Comments
Obstructive lung disease			
Common			
2. Chronic bronchitis	Fever	0–1	Acute exacerbations (i.e., respiratory infections) are accompanied by low-grade fevers not associated with chills or rigor. Nightsweats is uncommon. Patients are afebrile between exacerbations.
Uncommon			
4. Bronchiectasis	Fever, chills	0–2 0–1	Recurrent respiratory infections with fever are common in these patients. Chills and nightsweats may be present depending on the infecting organism. Some febrile episodes are related to mucus plugging of the airways.

Disease	Specific complaint	Severity	Comments
5. Cystic fibrosis	Fever, chills	0–2 0–1	Symptoms are similar to those described in bronchiectasis but occur at a younger age.
6. Upper airway obstruction	Fever	0–1	Fever does not occur unless the obstruction is related to an infectious process such as a peritonsillar abscess or necrotizing carcinoma.

Restrictive lung disease

Common

Disease	Specific complaint	Severity	Comments
7. Interstitial fibrosis	Fever, chills, nightsweats	0–3 0–3 0–2	Fever, chills, and nightsweats are unusual in patients with chronic disease. In patients with the Hammond–Rich syndrome (acute interstitial fibrosis), hectic fevers, chills, and nightsweats are common. Fever is common when the interstitial fibrosis results from lupus erythematosis or rheumatoid arthritis.
8. Sarcoidosis	Fever, nightsweats	0–1 0–1	Fever and nightsweats are uncommon except in patients who present with arthralgias and erythema nodosum.
9. Pulmonary edema	Fever, chills, nightsweats	0–3 0–3 0–3	Chills, rigor, and spiking temperatures are common in patients with noncardiogenic pulmonary edema secondary to sepsis or trauma.
10. Thoracic cage deformities and abnormalities	Fever, chills	0–2 0–1	Fever and chills are not due to the primary disease process, but are present during bacterial pneumonias that complicate the disease's chronic course.
11. Neuromuscular disorders	Fever	0–2	Patients with acute poliomyelitis experience low to moderate fever. These patients are prone to aspiration pneumonia, which is the most common cause of fever.

Disease	Specific complaint	Severity	Comments
12. Inhalational or occupational pulmonary disease	Fever, nightsweats	0–2 0–1	Coal miners' pneumoconiosis and silicosis are not associated with fever unless complicated by secondary infections. Patients with silicosis are at high risk of developing typical or atypical tuberculosis. The inhalation of nitrogen dioxide or phosgene may cause bronchiolitis obliterans with chronic fevers.
Uncommon			
13. Hypersensitivity pneumonitis	Fever, chills, nightsweats	1–3 1–2 1–2	Fever and chills may be a chief complaint. Patients acutely exposed to large amounts of the offending organism present with symptoms suggestive of pneumonia (e.g., fever, chills, and dyspnea). Characteristically, the fever occurs 4 to 6 hours after exposure and resolves spontaneously within 24–48 hours. Low-level chronic exposure to the same organisms is not associated with fever.
14. Goodpasture's syndrome	Fever	0–1	Fever is uncommon but may be related to the disease process itself, an inflammatory response to the intrapulmonary hemorrhage, or to secondary pulmonary infections.
15. Idiopathic pulmonary hemosiderosis	Fever	0–1	Identical to Goodpasture's syndrome.
Pulmonary vascular disease			
Common			
17. Acute pulmonary embolism	Fever, chills	0–2 0–1	Two thirds of these patients have oral temperatures higher than 100.4°F. Temperatures are occasionally as high as 102°F and may be accompanied by chills. The fever usually resolves within 72 hours.

Disease	Specific complaint	Severity	Comments
18. Sickle cell disease	Fever	0–2	Fever is common and may be related to pulmonary infarction and pneumonias or the nonpulmonary manifestations of this disease.

Tumors of the lung, pleura, and mediastinum

Common

22. Carcinoma of the lung	Fever, chills, nightsweats	0–2 0–1 0–1	Twenty percent of these patients present with fever, usually related to bronchial obstruction with a distal pneumonia. Tumor necrosis can cause fever.

Uncommon

23. Bronchial adenoma	Fever	0–1	Fever is an integral part of the typical clinical picture of the carcinoid syndrome. The fever is periodic.

Infectious diseases of the lung

Common

26. Bacterial, mycoplasmal, and rickettsial pneumonias	Fever, chills, nightsweats	0–3 0–3 0–2	Fever and chills may be a chief complaint. Single or repeated chills with fever may herald the onset of pneumococcal pneumonia. Bed-shaking chills are common. The fever, which fluctuates from 100°F to 104°F, returns to normal within 48 hours of administration of appropriate antibiotics. Repeated attacks of chills later in the course of the disease is suggestive of a nonpulmonary focus of infection such as meningitis, endocarditis, empyema, or arthritis. Fever and chills are also common in other types of bacterial pneumonia. Chills; the rapidity of the fever rise; the absolute body temperature; and the

Disease	Specific complaint	Severity	Comments
			duration, pattern, or resolution provide no diagnostic information about the etiologic agent in bacterial pneumonias. Patients with rickettsial pneumonias experience chills, sweats, and fever that may last for days to weeks. The pulse rate may not increase in proportion to the elevated temperature in these pneumonias.
27. Viral pneumonias	Fever, nightsweats	0–2 0–1	Chilliness as opposed to true chills may be experienced as fever develops. Although the absolute level of temperature elevation tends to be less than with bacterial pneumonias, this distinction is not clinically useful. The onset of fever is not as abrupt as in bacterial pneumonias.
28. Lung abscess	Fever, chills, nightsweats	1–3 1–3 1–2	Spiking fever and chills are common. They may be the main complaints, and their presence may be prolonged even with appropriate therapy.
29. Tuberculosis	Fever, chills, nightsweats	1–2 0–1 1–3	Fever begins gradually. Many patients are unaware of the increased temperature until the onset of nightsweats. A patient occasionally presents with high spiking fevers, suggestive of a concomittant bacterial pneumonia or endobronchial pneumonic spread of the tuberculosis.
Uncommon			
30. Atypical tuberculosis	Fever, chills, nightsweats	1–2 0–1 1–2	Fevers are similar to those in patients with tuberculosis.

Disease	Specific complaint	Severity	Comments
31. *Actinomyces* and *Nocardia*	Fever, chills, nightsweats	1–2 0–1 0–1	Prolonged and indolent fevers are common in these diseases; Chills are occasionally present.
32. Mycoses	Fever, nightsweats	1–2 1–3	Prolonged fever is common and may be a chief complaint. There may be exaggerated swings in the normal diurnal temperature variation with fever beginning late in the evening. Nightsweats are common; chills are distinctly unusual.
Miscellaneous			
34. Aspiration lung diseases	Fever, chills, nightsweats	1–2 0–1 0–1	Aspiration of acid gastric content causes acute chemical pneumonitis that may be accompanied by fever up to 102°F (39°C). Bacterial infections may complicate aspirations, but they are not required for development of fever. Chills can occur but nightsweats are more common. Aspiration of oral pharyngeal bacterial organisms causes bacterial pneumonia with fever, chills, and nightsweats. Foreign body aspiration can lead to fevers from post obstructive pneumonia.
35. Pulmonary alveolar proteinosis	Fever	1–2	Fifty percent of patients experience fever at some time during the course of the disease. The fever is thought to be related to secondary infections, but the cause is often not found.
36. Wegener's granulomatosis, its variants, and other vasculitides	Fever, chills, nightsweats	1–2 0–1 0–1	Fever can be caused by infection of the nasal–maxillary sinuses. Any of the diffuse vasculitides can be associated with fever.

REFERENCES

1. Atkins E, Bodel P: Fever. N Engl J Med 286:27, 1972
2. Dinarello CA, Wolff SM: Pathogenesis of fever in man. N Engl J Med 298:607, 1978
3. Murphy PA: Temperature regulation and the pathogenesis of fever. In Mandell GE, Douglas RG, Bennett JE (eds): Principles and Practice of Infectious Diseases, pp 399–406. New York, Wiley Medical Publishers, 1979
4. Patterson PY: Fever. In Youmans GP, Patterson PY, Sommers HM (eds): The Biologic and Clinical Basis of Infectious Disease, pp 97–105. Philadelphia, WB Saunders, 1980
5. Shulman JA, Schlossberg D: Fever and chills. In Walker HK, Hall WD, Hurst JW (eds): Clinical Methods, pp 29–32. Boston, Butterworths, 1976
6. Elin BJ, Wolff SM: Biology of endotoxin. Annu Rev Med 27:127, 1976
7. Dinarello CA, Goldin NP, Wolff SM: Demonstration and characterization of two distinct human leukocytic pyrogens. J Exp Med 139:1369, 1974
8. Bodel P: Pyrogen release in vitro by lymphoid tissue from patients with Hodgkin's Disease. Yale J Biol Med 47:101, 1974
9. Chao P, Francis L, Atkins E: The release of an endogenous pyrogen from guinea pig leukocytes in vitro. A new model for investigating the role of lymphocytes in fevers induced by antigen in hosts with delayed hypersensitivity. J Exp Med 145:1288, 1977

10 · MUSCULOSKELETAL AND DERMATOLOGIC MANIFESTATIONS OF PULMONARY DISEASE

ALBERT M. MARLAND

Definition
Mechanisms
Differential Diagnosis
Musculoskeletal and Dermatologic Manifestations in
     Specific Pulmonary Diseases

DEFINITION

Musculoskeletal manifestations of pulmonary disease include joint pain, myalgias, and finger swelling. Joint pain can be defined as arthritis—pain localized to the joint alone; arthralgias—pain felt in the joint with no objective or pathologic findings; periarticular pain—joint discomfort with pathological involvement of periarticular structures (bursae, tendons, bones); or referred pain—discomfort experienced both in distant structures and in the joints themselves.

Myalgia refers to musculoskeletal pain that may or may not be accompanied by objective physical findings in the affected areas. The pain can be present on movement or at rest and can be diffuse or limited to specific muscle groups (e.g., proximal muscles of upper or lower extremities). Weakness secondary to pain or muscular involvement by the primary disease (e.g., polymyositis) often accompanies myalgia. Myalgias are found in patients with primary lung diseases (viral pneumonias, sarcoidosis, primary lung carcinomas) or systemic diseases that affect the lung (polymyositis, systemic lupus erythematosus).

Finger swelling refers to articular, periarticular, periungual, and terminal phalangeal enlargement. Soft tissue enlargement is usually painless, while joint enlargement may be painful. Enlargement can be due to infiltrative diseases (clubbing; see Chap. 20), inflammation (rheumatoid arthritis), or edema.

The majority of dermatologic manifestations of pulmonary disease are caused by systemic diseases with pulmonary involvement as part of their multiorgan distribution. Skin lesions vary widely in appearance and diagnostic specificity.[1-3]

MECHANISMS

Most musculoskeletal manifestations of pulmonary disease are associated with multisystemic disorders that include the lung as a target organ. The collagen vascular diseases and vasculitides account for nearly all of these disorders.[4-11] The collagen vascular diseases probably arise from and are sustained by defects in the host's immune system. Rheumatoid arthritis typifies the pathologic finding in these disorders. An initial inflammatory and destructive event results in erosive synovitis. Release of inflammatory mediators, such as complement or kinins, increases the local tissue destruction. Cycles of inflammatory injury recur, causing further tissue destruction.

Many disorders do not fit this well-accepted pathophysiologic picture. The etiology of joint symptoms from pulmonary hypertrophic osteoarthropathy eludes definition (see Chap. 20). The causes of arthralgias and myalgias in bacterial infections similarly remain a mystery. Amyloidosis is an infiltrative disease with little or no inflammatory component.

Dermal manifestations of pulmonary disease may reflect the same pathologic process that affects other organs.[1-3] For example, necrobiotic nodules found in rheumatoid arthritis can involve both the skin and the lungs and are pathologically indistinguishable. Similarly, cutaneous abscesses from infection or vasculitic ulcers from systemic lupus erythematosus and other vasculitides can affect a multitude of organs including the skin and the lungs. In addition, the skin may react in a nonspecific immunological fashion to systemic diseases. Erythema nodosum can therefore occur in such diverse diseases as sarcoidosis, tuberculosis, coccidioidomycosis and *Mycoplasma pneumoniae* infection.[1,2]

DIFFERENTIAL DIAGNOSIS

Articular pain is precisely located, and movement of the affected joint is painful through all ranges of motion. Palpation of the joint structure produces pain. In contrast, periarticular pain is diffuse, and only specific joint movement in one direction produces pain. Palpation of the joint proper causes no discomfort. Referred pain is usually diffuse. Movement or palpation of the referring area produces pain in the distant location.

Monoarticular joint involvement suggests neoplasm; septic involvement from bacteria, fungi, or mycobacteria; rheumatoid arthritis; and rarely hypertrophic osteoarthropathy (see Chap. 20). Pyogenic involvement of the sternoclavicular joint is common in patients with intravenous drug abuse.

Polyarticular pain is less specific diagnostically than monoarticular pain.[4-12] Rheumatoid arthritis, systemic lupus erythematosus, and scleroderma produce symmetrical involvement of proximal large joints; in contrast, when ankylosing spondylitis affects nonaxial joints, asymmetry is common.[13] Systemic disorders such as viral diseases, bacterial endocarditis, and immune complex disorders (serum sickness or hypersensitivity pneumonitis) tend to involve large and small joints diffusely.[14]

Up to 50% of patients with polymyositis have muscle pain or tenderness.[10] Proximal muscles are more commonly involved than distal muscles. Myalgias are also associated with a multitude of other pulmonary and nonpulmonary diseases.

MUSCULOSKELETAL AND DERMATOLOGIC MANIFESTATIONS IN SPECIFIC PULMONARY DISEASES

The following table lists the musculoskeletal and dermatological manifestations in specific pulmonary diseases. The severity of the musculoskeletal complaints is classified as follows: 0 means no musculoskeletal complaints; 1 is mild—musculoskeletal pain, tenderness, limitation or aching only with exercise; 2 is moderate—musculoskeletal pain, tenderness, aching, or limitation with exercise and at rest; 3 is severe—chief complaint is limited activity due to severe musculoskeletal pain, aching, and tenderness that is present most of the time. The severity of the dermatologic manifestations is classified as follows: 0 means no dermatologic manifestations; 1 is mild (localized skin involvement); 2 is moderate (diffuse skin involvement); 3 is severe (diffuse skin involvement with symptoms, such as pain, weeping, burning, paraesthesias, etc).

| Disease | Complaint and severity | | Comments |
	Musculo-skeletal	Dermato-logic	
Restrictive lung disease			
Common			
7. Interstitial fibrosis	1	0	Myalgias and arthralgias are uncommon in patients with *usual interstitial pneumonitis.* Arthritis does not occur.
	1–3	1–2	Myalgias may precede by weeks or months the development of typical joint involvement in *rheumatoid arthritis.* Pain and swelling affect large peripheral joints in a symmetrical fashion. Skin lesions are rarely the initial complaint but are present in moderate to severe cases and tend to parallel the disease course. Rheumatoid nodules are found on the extensor surfaces of the extremities and the sclera. Necrotic vasculitic ulcers and digital microinfarcts are located in the distal lower extremities and the nail edge of the digital pulp respectively.
	1–3	1–2	Joint pain and swelling are the usual presenting complaints in patients with *systemic lupus erythematosus* and are indistinguishable from that found in patients with rheumatoid arthritis. A butterfly skin rash that worsens with sun exposure and Raynaud's phenomena are commonly present throughout the disease process. Necrotic leg or malleolar ulcers and periungal telangiectasia are occasionally found.
	1–2	1–3	Rheumatoid arthritislike syndromes; Raynaud's phenomena; erythema, swelling, and tenderness of the fingers; and intolerance to cold are common complaints in patients with *progressive systemic sclerosis.*

Disease	Complaint and severity		Comments
	Musculo-skeletal	Dermato-logic	
	1–2	1–3	Joint symptoms characteristic of rheumatoid arthritis, a rash resembling that of lupus erythematosus and polymyositis, Raynaud's phenomena, proximal muscle weakness, and myalgias may be present at times during the disease course. In patients with *mixed connective tissue disease*, a deforming arthritis similar to that of lupus erythematosus is not uncommon.
	1–3	1–3	Proximal muscle pain, weakness, joint pain, and deformity are common in patients with *polymyositis*. Patients with *dermatomyositis* suffer from myalgias. A characteristic lilac-colored rash involving the eyelids, bridge of the nose, cheeks, forehead, nailbed, and extensor joint surfaces may also be present.
8. Sarcoidosis	1–2	1–3	Arthralgias and myalgias are found in patients with erythema nodosum and chronic periarticular induration. Sarcoidal muscle involvement may cause mild to severe pain. Lupus pernio and vasculitic ulcers are frequently found in patients with advanced disease. Flesh-colored waxy papules, nodules, and plaques are found around the eyes and nasal labial folds.
10. Thoracic cage deformities and abnormalities	1–3	1	One third of patients with ankylosing spondylitis experience the early onset of peripheral arthritis. Lower back pain radiating no further than the knees and decreased spinal mobility are common initial complaints.

Disease	Complaint and severity		Comments
	Musculo-skeletal	Dermato-logic	
Uncommon			
13. Hypersensitivity pneumonitis	1–2	0	Arthralgias and myalgias are common in patients with acute hypersensitivity pneumonitis.
Pulmonary vascular diseases			
Uncommon			
18. Sickle cell disease	1–3	0	Back and knee pain and joint swelling are common and recurrent complaints of patients with this disorder. Joint effusions abate as the sickle cell crisis resolves.
Tumors of the lung, pleura, and mediastinum			
Common			
22. Carcinoma of the lung	1–3	1–3	Painful swollen joints and fingers (see Chap. 20), flushing, and alterations in skin pigmentation occur in patients with primary carcinoma of the lung. Skin metastases are uncommon. Ten percent of all acanthosis nigricans cases are associated with bronchogenic carcinoma. Because carcinoma of the lung can metastasize to bone, pain in the extremities, pelvis, or ribs is not uncommon.
Infectious diseases of the lung			
Common			
26. Bacterial, mycoplasmal, rickettsial pneumonias	1–2	1–2	In a small percentage of patients, bacteremia with seeding causes swollen, tender, and hot joints. Joint effusions and embolic skin lesions may be present. Erythema nodosum, erythema multiforme, pityriasis rosea, petechiae, mobilliform rash, and mucocutaneous ulcerations occur in 25% of patients with mycoplasmal pneumonia.

REFERENCES

1. Braverman IM: Skin Signs of Systemic Disease. Philadelphia, W B Saunders, 1970
2. Fishman AP: Pulmonary Diseases and Disorders. New York, McGraw-Hill, 1980
3. MacBryde CM, Blacklow RS: Signs and Symptoms. Applied Pathologic Physiology and Clinical Interpretation. Philadelphia, J B Lippincott, 1970
4. Rodnan GP: Primer on the rheumatic diseases. JAMA (Suppl) 224:5, 1973
5. Walker WC, Wright V: Pulmonary lesions and rheumatoid arthritis. Medicine 47:501, 1968
6. Gibson GJ, Edmonds JP, Hughes GRV: Diaphragm function and lung involvement in systemic lupus erythematosis. Am J Med 63:926, 1977
7. Gross M, Esterly JR, Earle RH: Pulmonary alterations in systemic lupus erythematosus. Am Rev Respir Dis 105:572, 1972
8. Hunninghake GW, Fauci AS: Pulmonary involvement in the collagen vascular diseases. Am Rev Respir Dis 119:471, 1979
9. Kelley W, Harris ED, Ruddy S et al: Textbook of Rheumatology. Philadelphia, W B Saunders, 1981
10. Bohan A, Peter JB: Polymyositis and dermatomyositis. New Engl J Med 292:344, 1975
11. Turner-Warwick M: Progressive airway obliteration in adults and its association with rheumatoid disease. Q J Med 46:427, 1977
12. Shaime OD: Cutaneous sarcoidosis: Clinical features and management. Chest 61:320, 1972
13. Rosenow EC III, Strimlaw CV, Muhm JR et al: Pleuropulmonary manifestations of ankylosing spondylitis. Mayo Clin Proc 52:641, 1977
14. Murray HW, Mason H, Sertefet LB et al: Protean manifestations of *Mycoplasma pneumoniae* infection in adults. Am J Med 58:229, 1975
15. Reynolds HY: Idiopathic pulmonary fibrosis. Clinical, histologic, radiographic, physiologic, scintigraphic, cytologic and biochemical aspects. Ann Intern Med 85:769, 1976

11 · HOARSENESS AND SNORING

KEVIN R. COOPER

HOARSENESS

Hoarseness or dysphonia is defined as a harsh or rough change in the usual quality of the voice. It usually indicates an abnormality of the vocal cord(s) and must be distinguished from other speech disorders. Dysarthria is a disturbance of articulation due to emotional stress or central nervous system disorders. Dyslalia is poor articulation due to structural defects or hearing loss. Dysphasia is a lack of speech coordination with failure to arrange words in an understandable way.

Mechanisms

Hoarseness is produced by disorders directly involving the larynx, which primarily functions as a sphincter, allowing air to enter the lungs but denying access to solid and liquid materials during swallowing. Secondary functions include phonation and laryngeal closure to allow for cough and straining.

The larynx is a complete arrangement of cartilage and muscle that controls the production of sound by modulating the movement of air as it passes through the vocal cords. Adductor muscles regulate the glottic opening, while abductor muscles increase and decrease its size. The lateral cricoarytenoid, the vocalis, the external thyroarytenoids, and the interarytenoids comprise the adductor muscle group and are opposed by the posterior cricoarytenoid muscle. These intrinsic laryngeal muscles are bilaterally symmetrical. They are ipsilaterally innervated by the recurrent laryngeal nerve with the exception of the interarytenoid muscle, which is innervated by both recurrent laryngeal nerves. Laryngeal nerve injury causes paralysis of both abductors and adductors muscles due to this innervation pattern.[1-4]

The cricothyroid muscle, an extrinsic pharyngeal muscle, tenses the vocal cords and is innervated by the superior laryngeal nerve, which is a branch of the vagus nerve. The right and left superior laryngeal nerves follow a similar course into the neck and divide into internal and external branches, innervating the upper and lower portion of the larynx respectively. After branching from the vagus in the neck, the right and left recurrent laryngeal nerves follow different courses to the larynx. The right recurrent laryngeal nerve passes under the right subclavian artery and then turns upward to the larynx. The left recurrent laryngeal nerve passes under the aortic arch before ascending to the larynx along the lateral wall of the trachea (Fig. 11–1). The course of this latter nerve makes it susceptible to damage by numerous intrathoracic pathological processes. Left vocal cord paralysis is an important

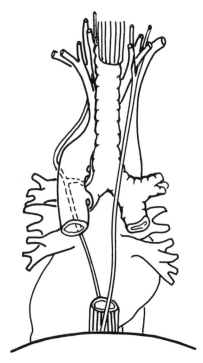

Fig. 11–1. Course of the right and left vagal nerves and the recurrent laryngeal nerve (posterior view). The left recurrent laryngeal nerve passes under the aortic arch before ascending to the larynx on the lateral wall of the trachea.

diagnostic clue suggesting the presence of an aortic aneurysm, an enlarged left atrium, a mediastinal neoplasm or lymphadenopathy.[5]

True vocal cord closure prevents aspiration but does not provide an airtight seal sufficient to withstand the pressures generated before coughing. Effective false cord closure is necessary for this seal. Midline vocal cord paralysis usually does not result in aspiration because the opposite normal cord is capable of crossing the midline to meet the paralyzed cord. Lateral (paramedian) vocal cord paralysis is associated with aspiration. Bilateral vocal cord paralysis will not lead to aspiration if the cords are paralyzed in adduction, but this position is associated with marked increases in airway resistance. Patients with bilateral midline vocal cord paralysis frequently experience severe dyspnea and are in danger of asphyxiation from upper airway obstruction.

Differential Diagnosis

Hoarseness is commonly experienced following overuse of the cords with prolonged shouting or cheering, upper respiratory infection, inhalation of irritant gases such as tobacco smoke, hot liquid ingestion, and administration of anticholinergic drugs. Vocal cord edema causes hoarseness in all these conditions.

Hoarseness may be due to vocal cord ulceration from continued placement of an endotracheal tube.[3,6] Ulcerations may also occur in tuberculosis, syphilis, typhoid fever, and lupus erythematosis. Vocal cord granulomas, papillomas, fibromas, and carcinomas may all produce hoarseness. Laryngeal carcinoma has an excellent cure rate primarily because a very small lesion produces hoarseness, permitting early detection.

Any condition(s) associated with generalized weakness such as myopathies, neuropathies, myasthenia gravis, botulism, hyperparathyroidism, and poliomyelitis may result in hoarseness. During thyroid surgery, vocal cord paralysis may occur from accidental trauma to the recurrent laryngeal nerves.[3,6] The most common cause of unilateral vocal cord paralysis is surgical trauma and other trauma followed by neoplasms and infections. Up to 40% of cases of unilateral vocal cord paralysis are idiopathic.

Bilateral vocal cord paralysis most often results from surgical trauma during thyroidectomy. Neurologic diseases are the second most frequent cause. Six percent of patients with bilateral paralysis have neoplasm. Many cases of bilateral paralysis are idiopathic.

SNORING

Snoring is defined as noisy breathing during sleep. A characteristic rattling inspiratory component may or may not be accompanied by expiratory sounds.[9] Snoring produced through the nose with the mouth closed (nasal snoring) is not pathological. Oral snoring (mouth open) implies partial upper airway obstruction.

Oral snoring is produced when air flow vibrates the relatively flaccid soft palate and the faucial pillars. The likelihood that snoring will develop is determined by both anatomic (the size of the upper airway and shape of the circumferential structures) and functional (muscle tone, edema, and body position) factors. During inspiration, hypopharyngeal pressures fall below atmospheric pressure, allowing air to enter the lungs. This pressure drop along with gravitational forces narrows the oropharynx, which is more pliable during sleep because of decreased muscle tone. Air passage through this narrow floppy passageway results in characteristic vibrations identified as snoring (Fig. 11–2).

Snoring is more common in deep sleep than in light sleep because of its dependence on decreased muscle tone; it occurs in REM sleep to approximately the same degree as in light sleep. In general, the louder the noise produced during inspiration, the more severe the upper airway narrowing.

The tongue makes up the greatest portion of the anterior wall of the hypopharynx. The supine position is most likely to produce snoring because the tongue is pulled back further into the pharynx.[9] Lying in the prone or lateral decubitus positions usually prevents snoring except in individuals with very severe upper airway narrowing.

Differential Diagnosis

It is uncertain whether snoring should be regarded as a consistent symptom of disease because nearly 10% of all people snore regularly. The frequency of snoring increases with age, weight, and ingestion of alcohol and sleeping pills and tends to be worse in men. Snoring may indicate partial obstruction of the upper airway, which can produce symptoms if severe enough. Snoring ceases if upper airway obstruction becomes complete, and the patient then experiences an apneic episode, defined as cessation of air flow for more than 10 to 15 seconds.

Virtually every patient with the obstructive sleep apnea syndrome snores. This condition is characterized by frequent apneic spells during sleep and is sometimes accompanied by pulmonary hypertension, right-sided heart failure, systemic hypertension, hypersomnolence, hypercapnea, personality changes, cyanosis, twitching movements during sleep, and polycythemia.[10,11] The basic mechanism of obstructive sleep apnea is cessation of breathing for periods of 10 to 90 seconds due to upper airway occlusion while asleep. These episodes can cause profound hypoxemia and disturbances of normal sleep

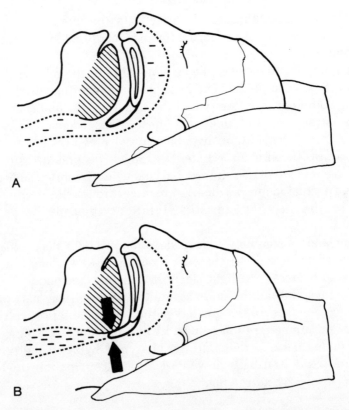

Fig. 11–2. Mechanisms for pharyngeal narrowing and snoring. *A*, During inspiration in the prone sleeping position, air flows into the trachea; during diaphragmatic descent, negative intranasal and intratracheal pressure is generated. The tongue (*oblique lines*) maintains its muscle tone and does not fall posteriorly in normal people. *B*, In patients with obstructive sleep apnea, the negative intratracheal and intranasal pressures cause the tongue to move posteriorly leading to partial or full occlusion. With partial occlusion, snoring ensues.

cycles. Arousal from deep sleep and reestablishment of ventilation are the only means of avoiding suffocation.

Obviously, many people who snore do not have the sleep apnea syndrome. In fact, when the apneic spell occurs, no sound is produced because there is no air movement. Many people have apneic spells during sleep without any detectable ill effects, but some effect on health is usually detectable when the apneic spells are particularly numerous and prolonged. There is no evidence that people who snore but experience no apneic spells suffer any adverse consequences.

It is important to distinguish snoring from other noises that occur during sleep, such as wheezing. Wheezing is predominantly an expiratory, high-pitched noise. Snoring is more rattling and is inspiratory.

HOARSENESS AND SNORING

Hoarseness and Snoring in Specific Pulmonary Diseases

The following table lists certain characteristics of hoarseness in relation to specific pulmonary diseases. Hoarseness can be classified as follows: 0 means it is not present; 1 is mild (a slight, almost unnoticeable change in voice); 2 is moderate (a definitive change in voice); and 3 is a definitive change of voice making speech difficult and words hard to recognize.

Snoring can be classified as follows: 0 means no snoring is present; 1 is mild (intermittent snoring that does not awaken the subject or sleeping partner); 2 is moderate (more continuous snoring that awakens the sleeping partner); and 3 is severe (continuous snoring that is very loud, keeps the partner awake, and often awakens the subject). If hoarseness or snoring is a chief complaint of a specific disease process, this is noted under Comments.

| Disease | Complaint and severity | | Comments |
	Hoarse-ness	Snoring	
Obstructive lung disease			
Common			
6. Upper airway obstruction	1–3	1	Hoarseness is frequently the chief complaint in the various diseases that cause upper airway obstruction. Hoarseness and upper airway obstruction in adults suggests bilateral vocal cord paralysis. Certain patients with upper airway obstruction may also experience the onset of snoring.
Restrictive lung disease			
Common			
8. Sarcoidosis	0–1	0	Although uncommon, noncaseating vocal cord granulomas may cause horseness.

Disease	Complaint and severity		Comments
	Hoarse-ness	Snoring	
9. Pulmonary edema	0–1	0	Rarely, left atrial dilatation can compress the recurrent laryngeal nerve.
12. Inhalational or occupational pulmonary disease	0–1	0	Hoarseness may follow inhalation of many types of dust, vapors, and fumes. The hoarseness is either due to a direct irritant effect, or possibly to drying of the upper respiratory tract mucosa.

Tumors of the lung, pleura, and mediastinum

Common

22. Carcinoma of the lung	1–3	0	Hoarseness may be the chief complaint in a small number of patients. Unilateral paralysis of the left vocal cord is a common finding in patients with lung carcinoma, implying that the cancer is not surgically resectable.
23. Metastatic carcinoma of the lung	1–2	0	Any tumor that metastasizes to the mediastinal lymph nodes may produce left vocal cord paralysis. Tumors of the prostate, gastrointestinal tract, and gonads are particularly likely to involve mediastinal lymph nodes.

Uncommon

24. Malignant mesothelioma	1–2	0	The pleural mediastinal surface may rarely be involved by this tumor, causing unilateral left vocal cord paralysis.

Disease	Complaint and severity		Comments
	Hoarse-ness	Snoring	

Infectious diseases of the lung

Common

26. Bacterial, rickettsial, and mycoplasmal pneumonias	1–2	0	Hoarseness occurs rarely with bacterial pneumonias and is due to direct irritation of the vocal cords by the infecting agent or as a result of the inflammatory response.
27. Viral pneumonias	1–2	0	Viral pneumonias occasionally cause hoarseness by direct irritation of the vocal cords or as a result of the inflammatory response.
29. Tuberculosis	1–3	0	Hoarseness is a common complaint in patients with tuberculous laryngitis, a very contagious form of tuberculosis. There is a relatively high incidence of tuberculous laryngitis and vocal cord ulceration in patients with long-standing advanced pulmonary tuberculosis. Laryngeal tuberculosis is rarely the only detectable sign of the tuberculous infection.

Uncommon

32. Mycoses	1–2	0	Pulmonary parenchymal infection may result in mediastinal adenopathy and damage to the left recurrent laryngeal nerve. Histoplasmosis can cause extensive mediastinal lymphadenopathy and fibrosis with subsequent trapping of the left recurrent laryngeal nerve.

| Disease | Complaint and severity | | Comments |
	Hoarse-ness	Snoring	
Miscellaneous			
34. Aspiration lung diseases	1–2	0	Impaction of a foreign body on the larynx or direct irritation of the vocal cords by the acid gastric content can cause hoarseness.
36. Wegener's granulomatosis, its variants, and other vasculitides	1–2	0	Because this disease is characterized by destructive granulomas in the upper airways, laryngeal involvement is common.
38. Sleep apnea and central hypoventilation syndrome	0	1–3	Snoring may be the chief complaint in patients with obstructive sleep apnea. Noisy breathing is experienced at night in patients with central sleep apnea.

REFERENCES

1. Proctor DF: The upper airways. II. The larynx and trachea. Am Rev Respir Dis 115:315, 1977
2. Paparella M, Shumrick D: Otolaryngology, Chaps 35, 36. Philadelphia, W B Saunders, 1980
3. Hedley–White J: Applied Physiology of Respiratory Care, p 3. Boston, Little, Brown & Co, 1976
4. Hyatt RE, Black LF: The flow–volume curve. A current perspective. Am Rev Respir Dis 107:191, 1973
5. Titche LL: Causes of recurrent laryngeal nerve paralysis. Arch Otolaryngol 102:259, 1976
6. Hedden M, Ersoz CJ, Donnelly WH et al: Laryngotracheal damage after prolonged use of orotracheal tubes in adults. JAMA 207:703, 1969
7. Weinstein L: Diseases of the upper respiratory tract. In Isselbacher KJ (ed): Harrison's Principles of Internal Medicine, 9th ed, pp 1254–1259. New York, McGraw-Hill, 1980
8. Pinals RS: Rheumatoid arthritis presenting with laryngeal obstruction. Br J Med 1:842, 1966
9. Lugaresi E, Coccagna G, Farnetti P: Snoring. Electroencephalogr Clin Neurophysiol 39:59, 1975
10. Guilleminault C, Tilkian A, Dement WC: The sleep apnea syndromes. Annu Rev Med 27:465, 1976
11. Block AJ: Sleep apnea, hypopnea and oxygen destruction in normal subjects: A strong male predominance. N Engl J Med 300:513, 1979

part II
SIGNS

12 · TACHYPNEA

BARBARA PHILLIPS

DEFINITION

Tachypnea is defined as rapid breathing associated with a respiratory rate greater than 20 breaths per minute. The normal rate in adults is between 14 and 20 breaths per minute.[1,2] Women tend to breathe more rapidly than men.

MECHANISMS

The respiratory rate is under both voluntary and automatic (involuntary or autonomic) control. The *involuntary* respiratory rate is a more meaningful indicator of the patient's physiologic status; it is therefore important to count respirations in a sleeping or distracted patient. While counting the respiratory rate, the physician can distract the patient by pretending to auscultate the abdomen.

The voluntary control system consists of the cerebral cortex, which modulates the respiratory rate through the brain stem and by direct transmission of nervous impulses to the respiratory muscles over the corticobulbar and corticospinal tracts.[3-5] The cortical control of respiration can override automatic control. This occurs infrequently except when the subject experiences pain, excitement, or anxiety.[2] Ondine's curse is a rare condition in which autonomic control of respiration is lost and voluntary control chronically predominates. This condition has been reported following bilateral cordotomies that interrupt the spinothalamic tracts.[3]

In contrast to the cerebral cortex, the brainstem regulates respiration automatically. Three respiratory centers located in the medulla and pons are primarily responsive to changes in Pco_2 and pH: the medullary center, which initiates and maintains inspiration and expiration; the apneustic center, which prolongs inspiratory effort and time (apneusis); and the pneumotaxic center, which helps to restrain the apneustic center.[3-5] These respiratory centers receive input from peripheral and central chemoreceptors, pulmonary and extrapulmonary receptors, and the cerebral cortex (Fig. 12–1).[4,5]

Carotid and aortic bodies are peripheral chemoreceptors that increase the respiratory rate by relaying nervous impulses through the ninth and tenth cranial nerves to the medulla. This occurs in response to a falling arterial oxygen tension. The peripheral chemoreceptors are stimulated whenever the PaO_2 is less than 500 torr, but are most active when the PaO_2 is between 30 and 100 torr. Nerve traffic from these chemoreceptors is actually suppressed at oxygen tension lower than 30 torr.[4,6] Ventilation increases by only 17% when these receptors are stimulated maximally at a PaO_2 of 40 torr.[2] Profound hypoxemia suppresses these receptors, and less profound hypoxemia stimulates them modestly. The respiratory rate is therefore an unreliable indicator of hypoxemia. There is a poorly defined central chemoreceptor located in the medulla that responds to changes in extracellular fluid pH in addition to peripheral chemoreceptors.[3]

Pulmonary receptors are identified as stretch receptors, irritant receptors, and J receptors. Stretch receptors inhibit inspiration during lung disten-

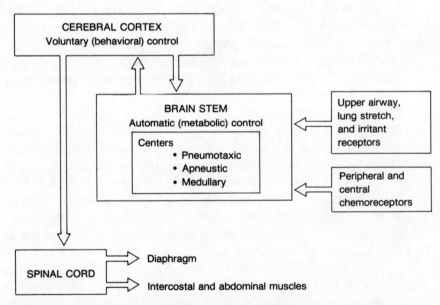

Fig. 12–1. Schematic representation of the respiratory control system, indicating the voluntary and autonomic control systems and the interrelation with mechanical receptors, chemoreceptors, and the spinal cord.

tion; irritant receptors are found among epithelial cells and are chemically stimulated to increase ventilation; and J receptors (juxta-pulmonary capillary receptors) are activated by increased pulmonary capillary volume or pressure. There may also be C receptors, which are stimulated by pulmonary congestion.[7] All pulmonary receptors transmit reflexes to the medulla through the vagus nerve.

A variety of other receptors and their associated reflexes, including those from the respiratory muscles, chest wall, carotid sinuses, aortic arch, pulmonary and coronary vessels, and somatic and visceral tissues, feed information into the respiratory center to control and modulate respiration.[3,4]

Changes in cerebral blood flow have a profound effect on ventilatory control. For example, cerebral hypoperfusion results in increased cerebrospinal fluid (CSF) Pco_2 and hydrogen ion concentration, causing hyperventilation.[3]

Arousal states also affect respiration. The respiratory rate decreases in slow wave sleep and becomes irregular in REM sleep.[8] Sleep depresses the ventilatory response to chemical stimuli. Many factors affect the rate, pattern, and amplitude of respiration. The final respiratory rate depends on integration of a variety of signals by the brainstem respiratory center.

TACHYPNEA IN PULMONARY DISORDERS

Tachypnea is thought to be mediated by receptors located in the chest wall, airways, the extrathoracic muscles of respiration and the diaphragm in patients with pulmonary diseases associated with lung hyperinflation and flat diaphragms (emphysema, bronchitis, and acute asthma).[9] Tachypnea is mediated in part by reflexes originating from the inflamed bronchial mucosal, intrabronchial, and parenchymal stretch receptors in patients with airway obstruction.[11] In addition, marked fluctuations in pleural pressures have also been implicated in the genesis of tachypnea.[10,11]

The typical respiratory pattern in patients with restrictive disease (interstitial fibrosis, pulmonary edema, and chest wall deformities) is characterized by increased rate and decreased tidal volume. This pattern results in an increase in minute ventilation and hypocapnea. Lung and chest wall compliance are reduced in these patients while physiological dead space is increased. Tachypnea is partially modulated by J receptors, which respond to changes in interstitial volume in patients with interstitial disease (edema, fibrosis).[7] Reflexes probably arise from thoracic cage receptors or diaphragmatic receptors in patients with restrictive disease secondary to thoracic cage and neuromuscular disorders.

The tachypnea associated with acute pulmonary embolism is mediated by pulmonary J receptors.[12] Bilateral vagotomies prevent the hyperventilation characteristic of this disease. A multitude of nonpulmonary disorders are associated with tachypnea.

Nonpulmonary Causes of Tachypnea

Cardiovascular
   Decreased cardiac output from any cause
   Right heart failure from any cause
   Congenital heart defects
   Acquired cardiac defects (*i.e.*, mitral and aortic insufficiency, ruptured interventricular septum)
   Peripheral vascular spasm
   Shock or hypotension from any cause
Metabolic
   Methemoglobinemia and sulfhemoglobinemia
   Extreme cold or heat
   Drugs (*e.g.*, salicylates, ammonium chloride, etc.)
   Anemia
   Alcohol withdrawal
   Fever
   Thyrotoxicosis
   Primary metabolic acidosis
Mechanical or Traumatic
   Brain trauma
   Tracheal obstruction (*i.e.*, croup, diptheria, pertussis, tracheomalacia, tracheoesophageal fistula, obstructed endotracheal tube)
   Abdominal distention
Miscellaneous
   Cirrhosis
   Amniotic fluid emboli
   Collagen vascular disease
   High-altitude residency

TACHYPNEA IN SPECIFIC PULMONARY DISEASES

The following table lists the presence and severity of dyspnea in specific pulmonary diseases. A positive (+) sign signifies that tachypnea is the chief finding in a specific disease; a positive/negative sign (±) means that the tachypnea *may be* the chief finding in a small percentage of these patients; and a negative (−) sign means that tachypnea may be present but *is not* the chief complaint. The severity of dyspnea is classified as follows: 0 means no tachypnea is present (respiratory rate is less than 20 breaths per minute); 1 is mild tachypnea (respiratory rate 20 to 25 breaths per minute); 2 is moderate (respiratory rate 25 to 30 breaths per minute); and 3 is severe (respiratory rate greater than 30 breaths per minute).

Diseases	Chief findings of tachypnea	Severity	Comments
Obstructive lung disease			
Common			
1. Emphysema	±	1–3	Tachypnea becomes more profound as the disease progresses. Respiratory rates of 25 to 30 breaths per minute are not uncommon in patients with advanced disease.
2. Chronic bronchitis	−	1–2	Tachypnea is usually less severe than in patients with emphysema. For reasons that are unclear, patients who eventually become hypercapneic have shallow and rapid respiration. Normocapneic patients with the same degree of lung function impairment maintain a relatively normal respiratory pattern.
3. Asthma	+	2–3	Tachypnea is common during acute attacks. A respiratory rate in excess of 30 breaths per minute is a poor prognostic sign.
Uncommon			
4. Bronchiectasis	−	1–3	Exacerbations of tachypnea occur during intercurrent infections, bronchospasm, hemoptysis, and pneumothorax.
5. Cystic fibrosis	−	2–3	Tachypnea becomes more severe as the disease progresses.

Diseases	Chief findings of tachypnea	Severity	Comments
6. Upper airway obstruction	−	1–3	Tachypnea is due to some combination of increased airway resistance with decreased air flow, hypoxemia, hypercapnea, or acidosis. Foreign body aspiration may cause tachypnea as a result of anxiety.

Restrictive lung disease

Common

7. Interstitial fibrosis	±	1–3	Tachypnea may be one of the earliest signs of interstitial fibrosis being noted before changes in the chest x-ray. Tachypnea worsens as the disease progresses. The decrease in tidal volume may lead to alveolar hypoventilation and hypercapnea.
8. Sarcoidosis	−	1–3	Tachypnea is present only with exercise in mild to moderate disease. Tachypnea is a consistent finding in advanced disease.
9. Pulmonary edema	+	1–3	Tachypnea is one of the earliest findings in both forms of pulmonary edema.
10. Thoracic cage deformities and abnormalities	±	1–3	Increasing tachypnea is associated with respiratory failure.
11. Neuromuscular disorders	±	1–3	Increasing tachypnea is associated with respiratory failure.
12. Inhalational or occupational pulmonary diseases	±	1–3	Tachypnea is a variable finding depending on the specific disease entity and the degree of pulmonary involvement. Tachypnea is common in patients with asbestosis or silicosis. In contrast, tachypnea is uncommon in patients with coal miner's pneumoconiosis. Severe tachypnea can be found in patients with advanced byssinosis.

Diseases	Chief findings of tachypnea	Severity	Comments
Uncommon			
13. Hypersensitivity pneumonitis	−	1–3	The acute form of this disease is associated with tachypnea 4 to 8 hours after exposure to the offending antigen. The tachypnea is due to some combination of a decreased lung compliance and increased airway obstruction. Chronic hypersensitivity pneumonitis causes an interstitial fibrosis that results in persistent tachypnea.
14. Goodpasture's syndrome	±	1–3	Tachypnea is common secondary to hypoxemia and decreased lung compliance.
15. Idiopathic pulmonary hemosiderosis	±	1–3	Similar to Goodpasture's syndrome.
16. Eosinophilic granuloma	±	1–3	Tachypnea is secondary to the decreased lung compliance. In addition, a sudden onset or increase in tachypnea is associated with spontaneous pneumothorax.
Pulmonary vascular disease			
Common			
17. Acute pulmonary embolism	+	2–3	The acute onset of tachypnea is the most common physical finding in patients with acute pulmonary emboli.[12]
Uncommon			
18. Sickle cell disease	±	1–3	Tachypnea may be due to the *in situ* thromboembolism, superimposed pneumonia, or progressive right heart failure.
19. Recurrent pulmonary thromboembolism	±	1–3	Tachypnea may be the most prominent finding.
20. Primary pulmonary hypertension	±	1–3	Tachypnea increases as the pulmonary hypertension worsens.

Diseases	Chief findings of tachypnea	Severity	Comments
21. Pulmonary veno-occlusive disease	±	1–3	Tachypnea is a common finding.
Tumors of the lung, pleura, and mediastinum			
Common			
22. Carcinoma of the lung	–	0–2	Tachypnea may be due to underlying chronic lung disease, pain, or lobar atelectasis. Patients with lymphangitic spread or diffuse alveolar cell carcinoma may have severe tachypnea.
23. Metastatic carcinoma of the lung	–	0–2	Tachypnea occurs in patients with pleuritis and pleural effusions from pleural tumor implants.
Uncommon			
24. Malignant mesothelioma	±	1–3	Tachypnea can be severe.
25. Bronchial adenoma	–	0–2	Tachypnea may be due to atelectasis or obstructive pneumonitis.
Infectious diseases of the lung			
Common			
26. Bacterial, mycoplasmal, and rickettsial pneumonias	±	1–3	Tachypnea is common in all forms of pneumonia and depends on the extent of lung involvement, associated chest pain, fever, anxiety, and hypoxemia. Patients with impending respiratory failure have respiratory rates greater than 30 to 35 breaths per minute.
27. Viral pneumonias	±	1–3	Tachypnea is less prominent compared to bacterial pneumonias.
28. Lung abscesses	±	1–3	Tachypnea depends on the size and extent of the abscesses.
29. Tuberculosis	±	1–3	Tachypnea depends on the extent of the tuberculous infection and the patient's underlying pulmonary reserve.

Diseases	Chief findings of tachypnea	Severity	Comments
Uncommon			
30. Atypical tuberculosis	±	1–3	Patients with *mycobacterium-avium intracellulari* disease may have progressive lung involvement and severe tachypnea.
31. *Actinomyces* and *Nocardia*	±	1–3	Tachypnea is common.
32. Mycoses	±	1–3	Tachypnea is common and depends on the extent of pulmonary parenchymal involvement, presence of pleural effusions, hypoxemia, and fever.
Miscellaneous			
34. Aspiration lung diseases	±	1–3	Tachypnea depends on the amount and type of material aspiration, its pH, and the degree of hypoxemia.
35. Pulmonary alveolar proteinosis	+	1–3	Progressive disabling tachypnea occurs in approximately two thirds of these patients. Tachypnea may worsen when secondary pulmonary infection supervenes.
36. Wegener's granulomatosis, its variants, and other vasculitides	±	1–3	As these diseases progress and diffusely involve the lung, tachypnea may worsen.

REFERENCES

1. DeGowin EL, DeGowin RL: Bedside Diagnostic Examination, p 265. London, MacMillan, 1970
2. Walker HK, Hall WD, Hurst JW et al: Clinical Methods. The History, Physical and Laboratory Examinations, p 430. Boston, Butterworths, 1976
3. Comroe JH: Physiology of Respiration, p 22. Chicago, Yearbook Medical Publishers, 1965
4. Mitchell RA: Neural regulations of respiration. In Williams MH (ed): Clinics of Chest Medicine—Disturbances of Respiratory Control, Vol 1, pp 3–13. Philadelphia, WB Saunders, 1980
5. Berger AJ, Mitchell RA, Severinghaus JW: Regulation of respiration. N Engl J Med 297:92–97, 138–143, 194–201, 1977
6. Fraser RG, Pare JAP: Diagnosis of Diseases of the Chest, Vol 3, p 1921. Philadelphia, WB Saunders, 1979

7. Kornbluth RS, Turino GM: Respiratory control in diffuse interstitial lung disease and diseases of the pulmonary vasculature. In Williams MH (ed): Clinics in Chest Medicine—Disturbances of Respiratory Control, p 91–102, Philadelphia, WB Saunders, 1980
8. Cherniack NS: Respiratory dysrhythmias during sleep. N Engl J Med 305:325, 1981
9. Park SS: Respiratory control in chronic obstructive pulmonary disease. In Williams MH (ed): Clinics in Chest Medicine—Disturbance of Respiratory Control, p 73. Philadelphia, WB Saunders, 1980
10. Grassino A, Sorli J, Lorange G: Respiratory drive and timing in chronic obstructive disease. Chest (Suppl) 73:290, 1978
11. Sant Ambrogia G, Miserocci A: Functional localization of the pulmonary stretch receptors in the airways of the cat. Arch Fisiol 70:3, 1974
12. Horres AD, Bernthal T: Localized multiple minute pulmonary embolism and breathing. J Appl Physiol 16:842, 1961

13 · MUSCLES OF RESPIRATION

R. CRYSTAL POLATTY

DEFINITION

The respiratory muscles include the diaphragm, intercostals, scalenes, sternocleidomastoids, and abdominals. These muscles generate the change in intrathoracic pressures necessary for ventilation (e.g., air movement into and out of the lungs). These muscles can be separated into inspiratory and expiratory and further subdivided into primary or accessory (Table 13–1). Certain muscles may function during both inspiration and expiration in conditions requiring maximal respiratory effort.[1-4]

MECHANISMS

Characteristics of Respiratory Muscles

When compared to other skeletal muscles, the respiratory muscles are unique in several respects: they are under voluntary and involuntary control, they must contract at frequent intervals in order to sustain life, and they must overcome elastic (as in pulmonary fibrosis) and resistive (as in obstructive airway disease) forces, whereas other skeletal muscles encounter only inertial forces.

Similar to other skeletal muscles, the force–length and the force–volume relationships of respiratory muscles are important in modifying contraction strength. In general, the longer the muscle length before contraction, the

Table 13–1. Classification of respiratory muscles by function

Function	Muscle
Inspiration	
Primary	Diaphragm
	External intercostals
Accessory	Scalenes
	Sternocleidomastoids
	Posterior neck muscles
	Trapezius
	Mylohyoids
	Pectoralis minor
	Muscles of the pharynx and face
	digastrics
	alae nasi
	platysmas
	facial cheek muscles
	levator palati
	laryngeal muscles
	tongue
Expiration	
Primary	Abdominal muscles
	external obliques
	rectus abdominus
	internal obliques
	transversus abdominus
Accessory	Internal intercostals
	Diaphragm

greater the force of the subsequent contraction. Maximum tension develops at a fiber length 5% to 10% above the natural resting length (Fig. 13–1), which for inspiratory muscles occurs at residual volume and for expiratory muscles at total lung capacity. Diseases associated with shortening or extreme lengthening of the respiratory muscles cause a decrease in the tension developed during contraction.[1-4]

Inspiration—Normal Function

The most important inspiratory muscles are the diaphragm (Fig. 13–2) and the external intercostals. Diaphragmatic slips arise from the second and third lumbar vertebra, the upper margin of the lower six ribs, and the

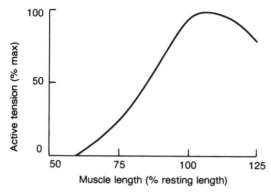

Fig. 13–1. Length–tension curve for a respiratory muscle. Maximum tension develops 5% to 10% above the natural resting muscle length (e.g., 100%).

xyphoid process. The diaphragm is innervated by the phrenic nerve, deriving fibers from the anterior nerve roots of C3 to C5.

Diaphragmatic descent decreases intrathoracic pressure, moving air into the lungs and causing chest expansion and compression of the abdominal contents. Thus, with inspiration the chest and abdomen expand at the same time. This is termed *synchronous breathing* (Fig. 13–3A). In addition, diaphragmatic contraction lifts and expands the rib cage, increasing the antero-posterior diameter of the chest. This is referred to as a "bucket handle" motion (Fig. 13–4A).

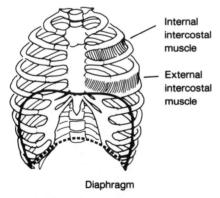

Fig. 13–2. Diaphragmatic structure. The diaphragm is the most important inspiratory muscle and arises from slips attached to the second and third lumbar vertebrae, the upper margin of the lower six ribs, and the xyphoid process. (——— indicates rest; – – – indicates inspiration)

The diaphragm is the only actively contracting muscle during quiet respiration in normal individuals. When respiratory demands are increased (exercise and acidemia) or when there is an abnormality of respiratory system structure or function, additional respiratory muscle groups contract.

Diaphragmatic excursion can be assessed by percussing the level of dullness between maximal inspiration and expiration, so-called tidal percussion. During inspiration, the level of dullness lowers due to diaphragmatic descent and the increased volume of resonant aerated lung. There is normally a 3 cm to 5 cm difference between maximal inspiratory and expiratory dullness.

The intercostals are the second most important inspiratory muscles. They are innervated by the intercostal nerves, which arise from the first

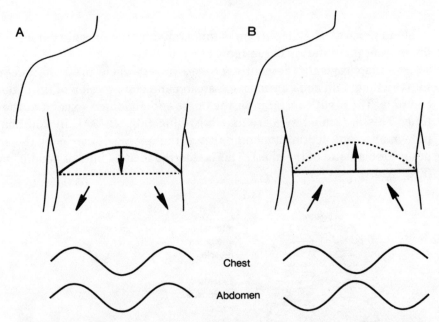

Fig. 13–3. A, Normal inspiratory function. The diaphragm descends (*arrows*), forcing the abdominal contents outward and resulting in *synchronous* movement as shown in the simultaneous tracing of chest and abdominal motion. B, Abnormal diaphragmatic movement. In patients with hyperinflated lungs and low, flat diaphragm (emphysema, asthma), the diaphragm no longer descends during inspiration; instead, the abdominal muscles contract causing the diaphragm to rise. The chest and abdominal movements are *asynchronous* because the chest expands while the abdomen moves inward and vice versa (*thoracoabdominal asynchrony*). (—— indicates rest; – – – indicates inspiration)

through the twelfth ventral thoracic nerve roots. The intercostal muscles elevate the rib cage and stabilize the chest by preventing inward rib cage motion, which facilitates maximal diaphragmatic excursion.

The scaleni and sternocleidomastoids are the accessory muscles of respiration that elevate and fix the first two ribs. They expand the rib cage and allow for better diaphragmatic length–tension relationships. The scaleni also expand the upper thorax; they are most active at larger lung volumes.

The sternocleidomastoids arise by two heads from the manubrium and the clavicle, fuse into a single belly, and insert into the mastoid process and occipital bone (Fig. 13–5). The sternocleidomastoid is innervated by the spinal accessory and second cervical nerves. The sternocleidomastoid increases the chest anteroposterior diameter by its action on the sternum. The sternocleidomastoids are active at tidal volumes of 2 liters or a maximum voluntary ventilation of 50 liters/min.

The laryngeal muscles, in addition to their role during phonation, allow air to easily enter and leave the chest. These muscles also protect the upper airway and help prevent aspiration.

Inspiration—Clinical Signs of Muscle Dysfunction

If the diaphragm is low and flat in the resting position as during hyperinflation from asthma and emphysema, several consequences may follow:[5]

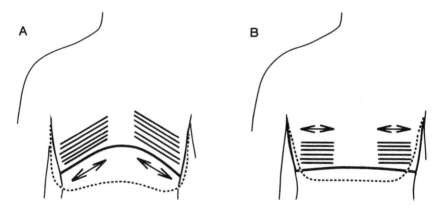

Fig. 13–4. A, The effect of normal diaphragmatic movement on the chest cage. As the diaphragm contracts and descends (*arrows*), the chest cage widens. B, The effect of abnormal diaphragmatic movement on the chest cage. Diaphragmatic contraction occurs in the horizontal plane (*arrows*) in patients with low, fixed diaphragms causing inward movement of the lower rib cage—Hoover's sign. (—— indicates rest; – – – indicates inspiration)

A   B

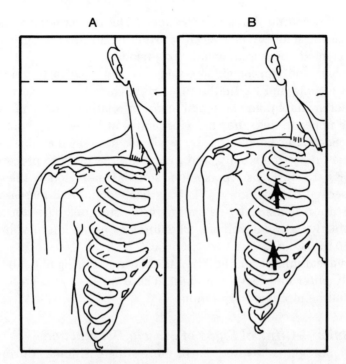

Fig. 13–5. The effect of sternocleidomastoid contraction on chest wall movement. A, The sternocleidomastoid arises by two heads from the manubrium and clavicles, fusing into a single muscle that inserts at the mastoid process and occipital bone. B, The sternocleidomastoid lifts the sternum increasing the chest anterioposterior diameter during active contraction.

1. The lower rib cage and costal margins may be drawn inward by the horizontal, inward shortening of muscular fibers during inspiration—Hoover's sign (Fig. 13–4B; compare with Fig. 13–4A).
2. Tidal percussion demonstrates little or no change in diaphragm position.
3. Inward motion of the abdominal wall may occur during inspiration and is paradoxical. This is called *thoracoabdominal asynchrony* (Fig. 13–3B), in contrast to *synchronous breathing* (Fig. 13–3A), in which the chest and abdomen simultaneously expand due to the downward motion of the diaphragm. Thoracoabdominal asynchrony results in ineffective ventilation and is a poor prognostic sign associated with a high mortality. It occurs in patients with respiratory muscle fatigue (e.g., diaphragmatic paralysis or hyper-

inflated lungs). Thoracoabdominal asynchrony is best observed with the patient in the upright position because gravity causes the diaphragm to be initially lower, thereby exaggerating the phenomenon in the patient with hyperinflation and a low resting diaphragm. The sign is more easily observed in the supine position in patients with pure muscle weakness or paralysis. Paralysis of one hemidiaphragm leads to decreased synchronous but not paradoxical motion.

4. The larger radius of a flat diaphragm compared to a domed diaphragm generates lower transdiaphragmatic pressures, leading to less effective ventilation with an increased work of breathing.

5. A downward movement of the trachea is caused by further descent of a low, flat diaphragm. This *tracheal tug* (Fig. 13–6) is due to the effect of the central diaphragmatic tendon attachment to the pericardium and other mediastinal structures.

6. Forced contraction of the abdominal muscles may push a low, flat diaphragm back into a more domed configuration improving its length–tension relationship. Such contractions can be palpated or observed at end inspiration. Diaphragmatic configuration also improves in the supine position because gravity allows the abdominal contents to move cephalad. These maneuvers can improve ventilation in the hyperinflated patient with chronic obstructive pulmonary disease (COPD).[6,7] The supine position may be deleterious

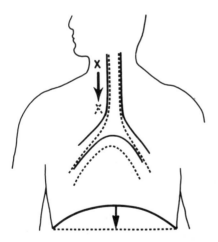

Fig. 13–6. Tracheal tug. Diaphragmatic descent in patients with low, fixed diaphragms causes downward movement of the trachea (*arrow*).

in patients with diaphragmatic paralysis because with inspiration the diaphragm is further "sucked" into the chest cavity.

7. Many emphysematous patients lean forward and elevate their rib cage improving diaphragmatic length-tension relationships.[8]

The intercostal muscles normally stabilize the chest wall and allow for rib cage expansion during inspiration. Paralysis of this muscle group leads to an inward motion of the rib cage during inspiration.[9,10] Inspection and palpation during this respiratory phase reveals an inward sucking of the intercostal spaces. In addition, intercostal muscle paralysis alters the elastic properties of the lung leading to alveolar collapse and a decrease in functional residual capacity and total lung capacity. The intercostals are not essential for continued ventilation unless the diaphragm is paralyzed.

Contraction of the scaleni, sternocleidomastoids, and other neck muscles is usually considered abnormal at rest (Table 13–2). The scaleni and sternocleidomastoid muscles hypertrophy in patients with emphysema. The sternocleidomastoids are particularly important in patients with chronic obstructive airway disease who have maximally fixed anteroposterior chest diameters because they facilitate an up-and-down movement of the fixed thorax (Fig. 13–5).

Expiration—Normal Function

Expiration is passive during quiet breathing. Potential energy is stored in the stretched elastic tissues of the thorax and lungs, allowing for recoil that is maximal at total lung capacity. Expiratory muscles are used at high ventilatory rates, during CO_2 breathing, or during maximal breathing maneuvers. The most important expiratory muscles are the abdominals, including the external and internal obliques, the rectus abdominus, and the transversus abdominus. Contraction of these muscles increases intra-abdominal pressure, causing an inward displacement of the abdominal contents and a decrease in

Table 13–2. Quantification of accessory muscle use

Designation	Amount of use
0	No accessory muscle use
1	Accessory muscle use determined by palpation only
2	Accessory muscle use just visible
3	Muscle use clearly visible
4	Sustained forced contractions

lung volume. Abdominal muscles start to contract at a minute ventilation of 40 liters/min to 50 liters/min. (normal, 5 liters/min to 6 liters/min). Full contraction occurs with coughing, straining, performing maximal maneuvers, or at a minute ventilation of 70 liters/min to 100 liters/min.

The internal intercostal muscles, including the interosseous and interchondrals, stabilize the chest wall during forced expiratory maneuvers, such as coughing, by moving the ribs downward. The scaleni also contract at maximal expiration, preventing the lung apices from herniating through Sibson's fascia. Scaleni contractions also oppose the downward motion of the upper ribs caused by abdominal contraction.

Expiration—Clinical Signs of Muscle Dysfunction

Palpation of the abdominal muscles should reveal no muscular contractions because normal expiration is largely passive. The presence of abdominal muscle contraction implies increased work of breathing because of increased ventilatory demands or abnormal respiratory system structure. Conversely, lack of abdominal muscle contractions during *forced* expiration may be a sign of muscular paralysis or weakness.

TESTS OF RESPIRATORY MUSCLE FUNCTION

A number of simple reproducible tests of respiratory muscle function help quantitate the degree of respiratory impairment and also measure the amount of respiratory reserve.[11]

The most important and objective technique for evaluating respiratory muscle strength is measurement of peak inspiratory and expiratory airway pressures. The device that measures these pressures is relatively unsophisticated, portable, cheap, and simple to use at the bedside. It consists of a mouthpiece, a one-way valve, tubing, and a pressure manometer in a closed system (Fig. 13–7). The patient seals his mouth over the mouthpiece, or the distal end of an endotracheal tube is attached to the apparatus. The peak expiratory pressure is measured by forced exhalation from total lung capacity, and the peak inspiratory pressure is by forced inhalation from residual volume. Respiratory muscle weakness, fatigue, and paralysis all cause a decrease in peak airway pressures (Table 13–3). The measurement of peak inspiratory pressures is important because inspiration is an active process requiring contraction of diaphragmatic muscles; however, measurement of peak expiratory pressures indirectly indicates the patient's ability to generate an effective cough or expectorate tracheobronchial secretions.

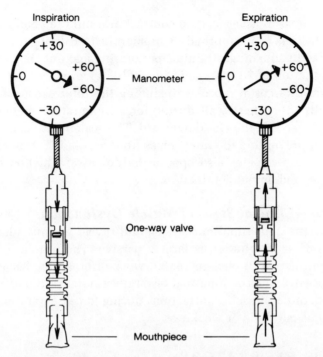

Fig. 13–7. Peak inspiratory/expiratory meter. To assess peak inspiratory pressure (PIP), have the patient exhale to residual volume, place his mouth tightly on the mouthpiece, and inspire as deeply as possible. In this example, peak inspiratory pressure is −60 cm H_2O. To assess peak expiratory pressure (PEP), have the patient inspire to total lung capacity, place his mouth tightly over the mouthpiece, and exhale as forcibly as possible. In this particular example, peak expiratory pressure is +60 cm H_2O.

A variety of other relatively simple tests may help assess the function of the respiratory muscles. These tests include measurements of the vital capacity, maximal voluntary ventilation, tidal volume, and arterial blood gases. Respiratory muscle strength, the presence of obstructive or restrictive lung disease, and the age, height and weight of the patient affect these tests (Table 13–3).[12]

More sophisticated tests include the following:

Electromyelogram (EMG). During contraction and relaxation, all muscle fibers undergo electrophysiological changes that can be measured and recorded by use of an electromyelogram. The "motor spikes" or electrical depolarizations are examined for their amplitude and velocity. A normal EMG is depicted in Figure 13–8. Muscle fatigue or weakness are associated with characteristic EMG changes.

Table 13-3. *Simple tests of respiratory muscle function*

Function	Normal	Respiratory* failure
Vital capacity (ml/kg)	65–75	<15
Tidal volume (ml/kg)	8–10	<5–7
Peak inspiratory pressure (cmH$_2$O)	−75–100	< −25
Peak expiratory pressure (cmH$_2$O)	>100	< +30–35

* Defined as PaCO_2 > 45 torr with low PaO_2

Fluoroscopy. There is normally as much as a 10-cm difference in the level of the diaphragm between maximal inspiration and expiration. The diaphragm is low during inspiration and moves high into the chest with expiration. The "sniff test" can be used to evaluate diaphragmatic function: in patients with paralyzed diaphragms, a sudden inspiration or sniff causes the affected diaphragm to move paradoxically at least 2 cm upward into the chest. Six percent of normal subjects have an abnormal sniff test.

Posteroanterior (PA) Chest Radiographs. Routine PA chest films show elevation of a paralyzed diaphragm. There may also be a shift of the mediastinum to the same side on inspiration.

Transdiaphragmatic Pressures (TDP). Pressures on both sides of the diaphragm can be measured to determine diaphragmatic power (Fig. 13–9). A normal TDP is 25 cm H$_2$O and does not exceed 6 cm H$_2$O with diaphragmatic paralysis.

Electrophrenic Stimulation. Electrical stimulation to measure conduction velocity can be performed on any peripheral nerve. The conduction time is slowed during certain disease states such as neuropathies. Phrenic nerve stimulation is somewhat more difficult to

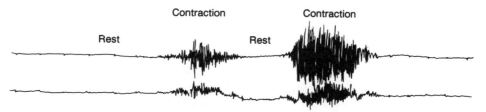

Fig. 13–8. Normal electromyographic tracing. Electrical activity is minimum at rest. During muscle contraction, activity increases as evidenced by increased amplitude and velocity of the electrical pulses.

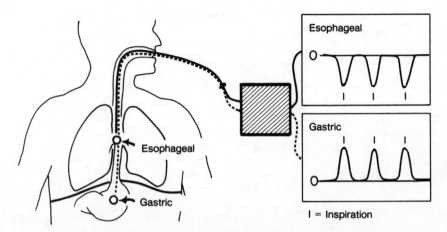

Fig. 13–9. Measurement of transdiaphragmatic pressures (TDP). TDP is the difference between gastric and esophageal pressure, measured either with two balloon catheters or with one catheter having two lumens and two balloons. One balloon is placed in the midesophagus to indirectly record intrathoracic pressure. The other balloon is placed in the stomach to record intraabdominal pressure. Gastric pressures normally rise with inspiration due to the descent and compression of the diaphragm on the gastric contents, while esophageal pressure falls, reflecting negative intrapleural pressures.

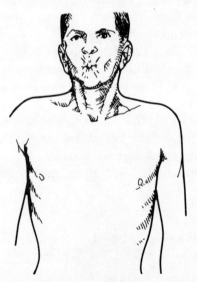

Fig. 13–10. Patient with advanced emphysema. This patient is purse-lip breathing during expiration. The sternocleidomastoid muscles are hypertrophied, weight loss is evident, intercostal space retraction is present, and the anterior posterior diameter of the chest is increased.

perform but can be helpful in determining whether the diaphragm is weak or paralyzed. The cause may be due to a central nervous system disorder, a primary phrenic nerve disease, or a muscular abnormality.

RESPIRATORY MUSCLE DYSFUNCTION IN SPECIFIC PULMONARY DISEASES

The following table lists the severity of respiratory muscle dysfunction in specific pulmonary diseases. The degree of severity is defined as follows: 0 means no respiratory muscle dysfunction; 1 is mild—respiratory muscle dysfunction is intermittently present and difficult to detect by physical examination; 2 is moderate—respiratory muscle dysfunction is continuously present and evident on physical examination; 3 is severe—respiratory muscle dysfunction is continuously present and is evident on casual inspection of the patient. The respiratory muscle dysfunction present in specific diseases is listed and discussed under Comments.

Disease	Severity of respiratory muscle dysfunction	Comments
Obstructive lung disease		
Common		
1. Emphysema	1–3	The low flat diaphragm is at a mechanical disadvantage, resulting in a decrease in peak inspiratory and expiratory pressures. Contraction and hypertrophy of the scaleni and sternocleidomastoid muscles, a tracheal tug, sucking in of the intercostal and supraclavicular areas, and forced expiratory abdominal muscle contractions are common with advanced disease. Hoover's sign and thoracoabdominal asynchrony are associated with a poor prognosis. The lips may also be used as an accessory expiratory muscle. Pursed lips act as a retard valve that maintains patency of the compliant or floppy airways (Fig. 13–10).

Disease	Severity of respiratory muscle dysfunction	Comments
2. Chronic bronchitis	1–2	Respiratory muscle dysfunction is less severe than in patients with advanced emphysema. The use of accessory muscles and decreased muscle pressures are common.
3. Asthma	0–3	No abnormalities of the respiratory muscles are found between attacks and during asymptomatic periods. Accessory muscle use is common during acute and severe attacks. Peak inspiratory pressures may actually be greater than normal due to the use of the accessory inspiratory muscles. Persistent contraction of the inspiratory muscles during expiration may account for some of the hyperinflation and prolonged expiratory flow times. Abdominal expiratory movements may be decreased. Thoracoabdominal synchrony is associated with severe airway obstruction.
Uncommon		
4. Bronchiectasis	1–2	Malnutrition, recurrent pulmonary infections, and weight loss can contribute to respiratory muscle dysfunction.
5. Cystic fibrosis	1–2	Pancreatic insufficiency, malnutrition, and cachexia, which are common in these patients, contribute to muscle weakness.
6. Upper airway obstruction	0–3	Complete upper airway obstruction causes all primary and accessory inspiratory muscles to contract forcibly without detectable air flow. Physical examination may reveal "sucking in" of the intercostal or supraclavicular spaces. Contraction of the sternocleidomastoids and scaleni allows the chest wall to expand even if there is no air movement. The expiratory muscles may contract forcibly in an effort to clear the airway.

Disease	Severity of respiratory muscle dysfunction	Comments
Restrictive lung disease		
Common		
7. Interstitial fibrosis	1–2	Peak inspiratory and expiratory pressures may be decreased.
8. Sarcoidosis	1–2	Sarcoid myopathies and neuropathies and myopathies secondary to steroid treatment rarely cause respiratory muscle weakness.
9. Pulmonary edema	1–3	Muscle weakness and fatigue in patients with cardiogenic pulmonary edema may be caused by a decrease in blood flow and oxygen delivery secondary to cardiac dysfunction, an increase in the work of breathing due to increased airway resistance or noncompliant lungs, and depletion of the short-lived diaphragmatic, intramuscular energy supply.
10. Thoracic cage deformities and abnormalities	1–2	In patients with kyphoscoliosis and thoracoplasty, costal versus diaphragmatic movement is restricted. Static muscle pressure is normal or supranormal, and there is experimental evidence that the diaphragm may actually be hypertrophied.
11. Neuromuscular disorders	1–2	Impaired chest wall motion can cause a decrease in minute ventilation and tidal volume in patients with Parkinson's disease. Patients with myasthenia gravis and Guillain–Barré syndrome have decreases in inspiratory and expiratory muscle pressures. Respiratory muscle weakness and paralysis may lead to respiratory failure in patients with poliomyelitis, amytrophic lateral sclerosis, and multiple sclerosis.
Uncommon		
13. Hypersensitivity pneumonitis	1–2	The use of inspiratory and expiratory muscles is common during the acute phase.

Disease	Severity of respiratory muscle dysfunction	Comments
Pulmonary vascular diseases		
Common		
17. Acute pulmonary embolism	0–3	Massive pulmonary embolism may be associated with the use of all inspiratory and expiratory accessory muscles.
Tumors of the lung, pleura, and mediastinum		
Common		
22. Carcinoma of the lung	0–3	Respiratory muscle abnormalities may be due to local tumor invasion of chest wall structures, metastases to the central nervous system, and paraneoplastic syndromes. Phrenic nerve involvement will cause ipsilateral diaphragmatic paralysis. There are several neurological syndromes associated with carcinoma that may induce muscle weakness including myalgias, the Eton Lambert syndrome, and carcinomatous myopathies.
23. Metastatic carcinoma of the lungs	0–2	Carcinomas occasionally metastasize to the diaphragm and the phrenic nerve. The generalized weight loss and weakness associated with metastatic carcinoma can also affect the respiratory muscles. Lymphangitic spread of certain carcinomas can lead to significant restrictive disease, dyspnea, and active recruitment of accessory muscles.
Uncommon		
24. Malignant mesothelioma	0–2	Respiratory muscle dysfunction may be due to a large pleural effusion or invasion of the chest wall and ribs.
Infectious disease of the lung		
Common		
26. Bacterial, mycoplasmal, and rickettsial pneumonias	0–3	Compliance decreases and hypoxemia ensues in patients with pneumonias that diffusely affect the lung. There is increased work of breathing resulting in recruitment of accessory muscles.

Disease	Severity of respiratory muscle dysfunction	Comments
27. Viral pneumonias	0–2	Similar to bacterial pneumonias.
28. Lung abscesses	0–2	Similar to bacterial pneumonias.
29. Tuberculosis	0–2	Cachexia can lead to respiratory muscle weakness and decreased muscle pressures.
Uncommon		
30. Atypical tuberculosis	0–2	Changes in respiratory muscle function are usually related to the underlying cystic or obstructive lung disease.
31. *Actinomyces* and *Nocardia*	0–2	
32. Mycoses	1–2	Diffuse mycotic pneumonias can lead to accessory muscle use and respiratory muscle fatigue.
Miscellaneous		
33. Aspiration lung disease	0–3	Bronchospasm and hyperinflation may occur with the aspiration of gastric contents. The respiratory muscle findings are similar to patients with asthma or obstructive lung diseases.
35. Wegener's granulomatosis, its variants, and other vasculitides	0–2	
36. Sleep apnea and central hypoventilation syndrome	0–1	Patients with central hypoventilation syndromes may have inspiratory muscle weakness.

REFERENCES

1. Campbell EJM, Agostoni E, Newsom–Davis JN: The Respiratory Muscles: Mechanics and Neural Control. Philadelphia, WB Saunders, 1970
2. Rochester DF, Braun NT: The respiratory muscles. Basics of Respiratory Disease 6, No. 4, March 1978
3. DeRenne J, Macklem PT, Roussos CH: The respiratory muscles: Mechanics, control, and pathophysiology. Part 1. Lung Disease: State of the Art, pp 255–269, 271–288, 289–309, August 1978
4. Sharp JT: Respiratory muscles: A review of old and newer concepts. Lung 157:185–199, 1980

 5. Shim, C: Motor disturbances of the diaphragm. Clin Chest Med 1, No. 1:125–129, 1980
 6. Ashutosh K, Gilbert R, Auchincloss JH et al: Asynchronous breathing movements in patients with chronic obstructive pulmonary disease. Chest 67:553, 1975
 7. Sharp JT, Goldberg NB, Druz WS et al: Thoracoabdominal motion in chronic obstructive pulmonary disease. Am Rev Respir Dis 115:47, 1977
 8. Gilbert R, Ashutosh K, Auchincloss JH, Jr: Clinical value of observation of chest and abdominal motion in patients with pulmonary emphysema. Am Rev Respir Dis 119:155–158, 1979
 9. DeTroyer A, Heilporn A: Respiratory mechanics in quadraplegia. The respiratory function of the intercostal muscles. Am Rev Respir Dis 122:591, 1980
10. Newsom–Davis J: The diaphragm and neuromuscular disease. Am Rev Respir Dis 119:115, 1979
11. Druz WS, Danon J, Fishman H et al: Approaches to assessing respiratory muscle function in respiratory disease. Am Rev Respir Dis 119:145, 1979
12. Rochester DF, Braun NMT, Arora NS: Respiratory strength in chronic obstructive pulmonary disease. Am Rev Respir Dis 119:151, 1979

14 · BREATH-GENERATED AND VOICE-GENERATED SOUNDS

CALVIN F. MORROW

R. PAUL FAIRMAN

DEFINITION

The two types of breath sounds possess characteristic qualities in normal individuals. *Bronchial* breath sounds are heard over the major airways and trachea, and *vesicular* sounds are heard over the remainder of the chest (Fig. 14–1).

CLASSIFICATION

Breath sounds in patients with pulmonary disorders can be classified as follows: decreased or absent, prolonged during the expiratory phase, or bronchial in an area where vesicular sounds are normally heard. Physical diagnosis is facilitated by evaluation of voice-generated vibrations to the chest wall, which may be identified by palpation or auscultation. These vibrations are described as normal, increased, or decreased in intensity.[1-3]

MECHANISMS

Sound Generation and Transmission

Considering the small volume of air and the low flow rates involved in normal tidal breathing, it is surprising that any sounds are generated during respiration. The vibrations produced are minute and have very low amplitude. Only the ear's remarkable sensitivity allows us to monitor these vibrations as sound.

Air flow is laminar (or streamlined) in the trachea and major conducting airways. Each layer of gas moves in a smooth path parallel to the walls of the airway, to be replaced by chaotic and turbulent flow in the more distal airways. Gas vibrations are generated within a frequency distribution of 200 Hz to 2000 Hz. The actual location of generated vibrations that produce the sounds heard through the chest wall remains uncertain. Most sound produced in the trachea and larynx is lost in transmission to the chest wall. At the other

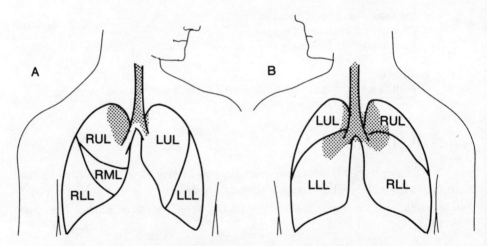

Fig. 14–1. Location of normal breath sounds. A, Anteriorly, bronchial breath sounds are heard over the trachea and the medial right upper lobe (RUL). Vesicular breath sounds are found over the rest of the lung. B, Posteriorly, bronchial breath sounds are present over the trachea, right upper lobe, and medial aspect of the left upper (LUL) and the left lower (LLL) lobes.

extreme, air flow in the terminal bronchioles and beyond is theoretically so slow that turbulence and therefore vibration and sound generation are unlikely, so breath sounds heard through the chest wall are dominated by those produced in the major airways.

Sound production also occurs during exhalation when the vocal cords are set into motion by the air stream. The result is the human voice, which is composed of complex frequencies ranging from 80 Hz to 10,000 Hz.

Sound Attenuation

Auscultation of the chest does not yield the full range of vibrations generated by tidal breathing or vocalization. This difference in sound content is due to the transmitting media, which include the conducting airways, lung parenchyma, pleura, and chest wall. As vibrations progress toward the periphery and through the chest wall, a variable amount of energy is lost, depending on the acoustic matching of the involved structures. The loss is slight in normal individuals but is increased by abnormalities in the pleural space (pneumothorax or hydrothorax) or pulmonary parenchyma (emphysema).

The lung and chest wall preferentially pass low frequency sounds, attenuate frequencies in the mid-range (200 Hz to 1000 Hz), and remove higher frequency vibrations (higher than 1000 Hz). This fact is important in the perception of voice sounds at the chest wall. Low, middle, and high frequency ranges are produced when vowels are vocalized. Each component frequency is required for comprehension of the vowel; therefore, the normal filtering of frequencies higher than 200 Hz renders speech in general and vowels in particular unintelligible at the chest wall.[1-3]

The mechanisms involved in sound attenuation include changes in the conducting medium and damping. Changes in conducting medium introduce resistance to transmission in the form of sound reflection. This acoustic impedence occurs at gas–liquid interfaces (e.g., in alveoli) and at the lung–pleura and pleura–chest wall interfaces. Damping occurs when a conducting medium is forced to vibrate at a frequency different from its natural resonant frequency. Damping of higher frequencies is maximal at the chest wall.

EXAMINATION OF THE CHEST

A reproducible approach during physical examination helps to identify any abnormalities. Observations are recorded both during shallow and deep breathing, and inspiration and expiration should be closely observed. The patients are used as their own control because of variable thickness and configuration of the lungs and chest wall. The sounds heard from one side of the chest are compared with those from a corresponding area on the opposite side. Considerable auscultatory experience with a wide range of normal breath sounds is necessary before abnormal sounds can be distinguished with confidence. Even when breath sounds at symmetrical sites on the thorax differ, it may be impossible to state which side is abnormal without the aid of a chest x-ray film. Symmetrical findings also may be misleading because similar pathologic processes may affect both sides (bilateral apical tuberculosis, causing symmetrical bronchial breath sounds). Nevertheless, comparison of one side to the other and the upper portion to the lower portion of the same lung is essential.[4]

NORMAL BREATH-GENERATED AND VOICE-GENERATED SOUNDS

Normal breath sounds have a characteristic quality that varies with the chest areas over which they are heard. Bronchial breath sounds are found over the large airways, (mainstem and some lobar bronchi; Fig. 14–1). These sounds are produced by vibrations extending from the threshold of human and auditory sensation to more than 2,000 Hz. Because these sounds are likened to those generated by air passing through a tube or the trachea, they are sometimes called tubular. The expiratory phase is louder, lasts about as long as the inspiratory phase, and is usually separated from inspiration by a short silent pause (Fig. 14–2).

Vesicular breath sounds are heard over most of the chest (Fig. 14–2). These are faint sounds within a frequency distribution between 200 Hz and 600 Hz. Inspiration is louder, higher pitched, and about three times the duration of the softer and lower-pitched expiratory sounds. The expiratory difference in bronchial (loud, prolonged) and vesicular (soft, short) breath sounds is characteristic (Fig. 14–2). In some areas of the lung, a clear distinction between bronchial and vesicular sounds cannot be made, and these intermediate sounds are referred to as bronchovesicular.[1–3]

Distribution and Characteristics

The terminology recommended by the American College of Chest Physicians for the sounds heard over the chest is normal, when they follow the characteristic pattern heard in normal persons. This normal pattern includes bronchial breath sounds over the trachea, the upper anterior chest both to the right and the left of the sternum, and posteriorly between the scapulae; and vesicular sounds elsewhere (Fig. 14–1). Deviation from this normal pattern suggests an abnormal underlying lung.[5,6]

The clarity and loudness of auscultated voice sounds at the chest depends on the loudness of the voice, its pitch, and the area of the chest examined. A loud sound results in greater vibrations being detected at the chest wall despite the normal attenuating mechanisms. Pitch becomes important if voice vibrations are controlled for loudness. A voice with fewer low frequency tones (about 200 Hz; as in women and children) will be transmitted less to the chest wall than one with more lower frequency tones as found in men.

A vowel sound will not be heard with clarity when auscultating the normal chest in areas where parenchyma overlie the airways. Its higher component frequencies are selectively filtered out, and the sounds lose much of the original sound intensity; however, in thoracic regions (e.g., over the right upper chest, sternum, and upper interscapular area) where the large airways are close to the chest wall, selective filtering is not fully exhibited.

Other chest areas in which voice transmission or clarity is improved or voice sounds decreased or absent are considered abnormal.

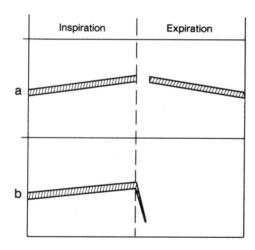

Fig. 14–2. Character and duration of bronchial and vesicular breath sounds. The duration and loudness of inspiration are similar in bronchial (a) and vesicular (b) breath sounds. In contrast, the expiratory phase of bronchial breath sounds is louder, lasts as long as the inspiratory phase, and is separated from inspiration by a short pause.

ABNORMAL BREATH-GENERATED AND VOICE-GENERATED SOUNDS

Decreased or Absent Sounds

A decrease in the intensity of breath and voice sounds results from increased thickness of the chest wall, decreased air flow to a segment of lung, hyperinflation of the lungs, and separation of the lung and chest wall by air or fluid in the pleural cavity.

When the chest wall is thicker than usual (fat or muscle), its filtering capacity increases and the intensity of breath sounds decreases. The diminished breath sounds found in obese or extremely muscular persons may become readily audible when the patient is asked to breathe more deeply.

Normal breath and voice sounds are generated by air flow in segmental or lobar bronchi. A major reduction or lack of air flow in an individual bronchus results in diminished or absent breath and voice sounds over the affected lung segment. Tumors, mucosal edema, mucus plugs, and foreign bodies can all reduce air flow sufficiently to decrease breath sounds.

Sound attenuation resulting from a mismatch in acoustic properties between the hyperinflated lung and the chest wall is best exemplified in patients with exacerbations of asthma in whom auscultatory breath sounds are often inaudible. Breath sounds return to their normal intensity with correction of the hyperinflation. In patients with emphysema, the gas and airway vibrations are already weak at their source and are reduced to silence by reflection at the lung–chest wall interface.

Normal breath-generated and voice-generated sounds are dampened by fluid within the pleural space. The attenuation is caused by sound reflection at the interface of media with widely different acoustic properties (lung and fluid, fluid and chest wall) and is not a result of poor sound transmission in fluid. A similar phenomenon accounts for the lack of breath sounds over a pneumothorax.[1-3]

Prolonged Expiratory Phase

The expiratory portion of a normal respiratory cycle is at most one third the duration of the inspiratory portion. Its duration is determined by the elastic recoil of the lung and the low resistance to air flow offered by the tracheobronchial tree. Alteration of these factors may change the duration of expiration. Reductions in expiratory time are clinically undetectable because expiration is normally quite short. Expiratory prolongation follows loss of lung elastic recoil (emphysema) or a generalized increase in airway resistance (chronic bronchitis or asthma).

Bronchial Breath Sounds and Increased
Voice Transmission

Bronchial breath sounds heard over portions of the chest where vesicular sounds are expected are considered abnormal. They result from the transmission of normal breath sounds with minimal high-frequency filtration by the lung. Consolidation (pneumonia, pulmonary edema), atelectasis, and extensive pulmonary fibrosis may cause this phenomenon. Bronchial breath sounds are generated in the airway supplying the consolidated lung. Vibrations are not generated, and breath sounds are decreased if the bronchus is not patent. An exception to this rule occurs in cases of upper-lobe bronchial obstruction. Over an airless upper lobe, bronchial breathing is often heard whether the bronchus is patent or obstructed because the mediastinal surface of the upper lobes is in contact with the trachea and sound is directly transmitted from the trachea to the lung, obviating the need for a patent bronchus.

Increased voice transmission is a result of the same processes that cause bronchial breathing (e.g., consolidation, atelectasis, and extensive parenchymal fibrosis). A number of older terms such as *egophony*, *pectoriloquy*, and *bronchophony* have been used to describe increased voice transmission. These terms are inappropriate because they apply to the same basic phenomenon.[5] A simple description of the findings as increased intensity or clarity of the whispered or spoken voice is sufficient. We define each term here because they are so frequently used.

When the selective filtering effect of the lung is suppressed, previously attenuated frequencies in the middle and high ranges become audible. The voice sounds will have a greater intensity (perceived as loudness) and clarity because the component frequencies have been restored. This phenomenon is called *bronchophony*.

Whispering normally produces only mid- and high-frequency vibrations. The majority of these tones are attenuated, and little sound is heard at the chest wall with an intact selective filter; however, these frequencies are transmitted when the selective filter is defeated. The sounds become clear and audible, which is a phenomenon defined as *whispered pectoriloquy*.

Loss of the selective filter from some pathologic process alters the transmitted quality of vowel sounds. The vowel "e" (as in he) is perceived as "a" (as in hay). This phenomenon is known as *egophony*.

SUMMARY

Abnormalities of voice-generated and breath-generated sounds parallel each other. Mechanisms that decrease the intensity of breath sounds also decrease the intensity of voice sounds. When pathological conditions result in bronchial breath sounds being heard over portions of the chest in which vesicular sounds are expected, increased voice transmission is apparent as well. Unfortunately, several pathological states may be responsible for either increased or decreased breath- and voice-generated sounds. Correlation with other physical examination techniques such as percussion (see Chap. 15) and adventitious (see Chap. 16) sounds may suggest a specific etiology.

Regional differences in anatomy and pathology may result in several abnormal findings in a single patient. For example, patients with cystic fibrosis often have decreased voice and breath sounds because of air flow obstruction. They may also have areas of consolidation with increased voice and breath sound transmission.

BREATH-GENERATED AND VOICE-GENERATED SOUNDS IN SPECIFIC PULMONARY DISEASES

The following table lists the most common characteristics of breath- and voice-generated sounds in specific pulmonary diseases. Breath and voice sounds may be classified as follows: N is normal; ↓ is decreased; ↑ is increased or bronchial. The expiratory phase can be classified as follows: + means prolongation consistently present; ± means prolongation may be present; and − means prolongation does not occur. Exceptions to these common findings are found under Comments.

Disease	Breath sounds	Voice sounds	Pro-longed expira-tory phase	Comments
Obstructive lung disease				
Common				
1. Emphysema	N or ↓	N or ↓	+	Patients with mild to moderate emphysema have no abnormal physical findings contrary to those with advanced disease.
2. Chronic bronchitis	N	N	+	The intensity of the breath sounds decreases during exacerbations of chronic bronchitis.

Disease	Breath sounds	Voice sounds	Prolonged expiratory phase	Comments
3. Asthma	N or ↓	N or ↓	+	Breath and voice sounds are normal between acute attacks. Breath and voice sounds decrease in intensity, and the expiratory phase prolongs as the severity of an attack increases. When airway obstruction is so severe that respiratory failure is imminent, there may be no breath or voice sounds. This is an ominous prognostic sign.

Uncommon

Disease	Breath sounds	Voice sounds	Prolonged expiratory phase	Comments
4. Bronchiectasis	N or ↓	N or ↓	+	Decreased breath sounds are heard in patients whose airways are occluded by secretions. Bronchial breath sounds are comon in patients with extensive, bibasilar bronchiectasis, peribronchial inflammation, and consolidation.
5. Cystic fibrosis	N or ↓	N or ↓	+	Similar to bronchiectasis.
6. Upper airway obstruction	N	N	+	Expiratory prolongation may be present in patients with intrathoracic or fixed upper airway obstruction.

Restrictive lung disease

Common

Disease	Breath sounds	Voice sounds	Prolonged expiratory phase	Comments
7. Interstitial fibrosis	N	N	−	Bronchial breath sounds are presumably caused by an increase in sound transmission through the abnormal lung. This is occasionally found in a patient with end-stage fibrosis.
8. Sarcoidosis	N	N	−	Patients with extensive fibrosis have bronchial breath sounds; patients with cystic disease have decreased sounds.

Disease	Breath sounds	Voice sounds	Pro- longed expira- tory phase	Comments
9. Pulmonary edema	N	N	–	Alveolar fluid filling and consolidation cause an increase in breath- and voice-generated sounds. Breath sounds are decreased in patients with pleural effusions. Bronchial mucosal edema may cause prolongation of the expiration phase.
10. Thoracic cage deformities and abnormalities	N	N	±	Airway compression with atelectasis causes bronchial breathing and increased sound transmission in patients with deforming kyphoscoliosis. Thoracoplasty with pleural thickening decreases breath and voice sounds. Marked deformity of the thoracic cage can "kink" the larger airways, causing prolongation of the expiratory phase.
11. Neuromuscular disorders	N or ↓	N or ↓	±	These findings are due to a decrease in tidal volume from muscle weakness.
12. Inhalational or occupational pulmonary diseases	N	N	±	Bronchial breathing may be present in patients with progressive massive fibrosis. Patients with diseases primarily affecting the airways have a prolonged expiratory phase and decreased sound transmission due to hyperinflation of the lung.
Uncommon				
13. Hypersensitivity pneumonitis	N	N	±	The alveolitis causes air space filling and an increased sound transmission. A prolonged expiratory phase is common in patients with clinically evident bronchospasm.

Disease	Breath sounds	Voice sounds	Prolonged expiratory phase	Comments
14. Goodpasture's syndrome	N or ↑	N or ↑	—	The alveolar filling process causes increased sound transmission.
15. Idiopathic pulmonary hemosiderosis	N or ↑	N or ↑		Similar to Goodpasture's syndrome.
16. Eosinophilic granuloma	N	N	—	An increase in voice- and breath-generated sounds may be due to end-stage pulmonary fibrosis. Pneumothoraces, which are a common complication, decrease sound transmission.

Pulmonary vascular disease

Common

17. Acute pulmonary embolism	N	N	±	Bronchial breath sounds and increased voice transmission occur in patients with pulmonary infarction and consolidation. Pleural effusions have the opposite effect. Clinically significant bronchospasm with prolongation of the expiratory phase is found in a small percentage of patients.

Uncommon

18. Sickle cell anemia	N	N	—	*In situ* thrombosis and pneumonias cause bronchial breath sounds, whereas pleural effusions decrease breath sounds.

Tumors of the lung, pleura, and mediastinum

Common

22. Carcinoma of the lung	N	N	±	Findings depend on the size and location of the tumor, bronchial impingement or obstruction, the presence of pleural effusions, post-obstructive pneumonias, and the extent of the underlying emphysema or chronic bronchitis.

Disease	Breath sounds	Voice sounds	Pro- longed expira -tory phase	Comments
24. Malignant mesothelioma	N or ↓	N or ↓	—	A thickened pleura decreases breath and voice transmission.
25. Bronchial adenomas	N	N	+	Breath and voice sounds decrease when atelectasis is present.

Infectious diseases of the lungs
Common

26. Bacterial, mycoplasmal, and rickettsial pneumonias	N	N	—	Bronchial breath sounds and increased voice transmission are common in consolidated pneumonias. Pleural effusions decrease both sounds.
27. Viral pneumonias	N	N	—	Small pleural effusions are common and decrease breath and voice generated sounds.
28. Lung abscesses	N	N	—	Physical findings depend on the extent of the parenchymal and pleural disease.
29. Tuberculosis	N	N	—	Findings depend on the extent of pulmonary involvement and the presence of consolidation and pleural effusions.

Uncommon

30. Atypical tuberculosis	N	N	—	Similar to tuberculosis.
32. Mycoses	N	N	—	Findings depend on the extent of pleural and parenchymal involvement.

Miscellaneous

34. Aspiration lung diseases	N	N	±	Findings depend on the presence of pulmonary consolidation or pleural effusion and airway obstruction with atelectasis. Aspiration causes prolongation of the expiratory phase secondary to bronchoconstriction.
35. Pulmonary alveolar proteinosis	N or ↑	N or ↑	—	Consolidation results in bronchial breath sounds.

REFERENCES

1. Murphy RLH, Holford SK: Lung Sounds. Basics of Respiratory Disease 8:1–6, 1980
2. Forgacs P: The functional basis of pulmonary sounds. Chest 73:399–405, 1978
3. Forgacs P: Lung Sounds, pp 26–44. London, Baillière Tindall, 1978
4. Crutcher JC: Chest auscultation. In Walker HK, Hall WD, Hurst JW (eds): Clinical Methods, pp 537–540. Woburn, MA, Butterworth Inc, 1976
5. Pulmonary terms and symbols: Report of the ACCP-ATS Joint Committee on Pulmonary Nomenclature. Chest 67:583–593, 1975
6. Leblanc P, Macklem PT, Ross WRD: Breath sounds and the distribution of pulmonary ventilation. Am Rev Respir Dis 102:10–16, 1970

15 · ADVENTITIOUS LUNG SOUNDS: CRACKLES AND WHEEZES

R. PAUL FAIRMAN

KEVIN R. COOPER

DEFINITION

Adventitious sounds indicate some abnormality of the pulmonary parenchyma or airways and are not found in normal persons. The major adventitial sounds are identified as crackles and wheezes.

Crackles, or crepitations, are discontinuous, interrupted explosive sounds with a wide spectrum of frequencies between 200 Hz and 2,000 Hz (Fig. 15–1A). The sounds may be high or low pitched, loud or faint, scanty or profuse. They are most often heard during inspiration but occasionally are found during expiration.[1-4]

Wheezes are continuous sounds with a musical character (Fig. 15–1B and C). Most of their sound frequencies are harmonically related, and the lowest frequency determines their pitch. Wheezes may be subclassified by their pitch, timing in the respiratory cycle, duration, and whether they are single or multiple.[1-4] Wheezes are predominantly expiratory. Stridor is a loud audible musical sound, similar to a wheeze, which is predominantly inspiratory in timing.

The *pleural rub* is an additionally grating adventitious sound unaffected by cough and heard during both inspiration and expiration.[2] The components of a pleural friction rub may be confused with the crackling sounds of pulmonary crackles because the acoustic properties of the two are quite similar.

TERMINOLOGY

For many decades adventitious sounds were called rales or rhonchi. Due to modern research, however, these terms are changing. Forgacs' landmark studies of lung sounds used wave form analysis.[1-3] Sounds were recorded and replayed on a greatly expanded time scale. Under these circumstances, each sound could be examined closely and its timing and frequency determined. From these studies, Forgacs recommended the terms *crackles* and *wheezes* rather than *rales* and *rhonchi*. He reasoned that the historical terms had no basis in acoustical physiology and that their meanings had become blurred by years of inaccurate use. The recommended terms were chosen because they could be defined by specific acoustic characteristics. These newer terms have not been accepted by all physicians, and uniform terminology may never be achieved; nevertheless, terms based on acoustic characteristics should permit more accurate communication between investigators and clinicians.

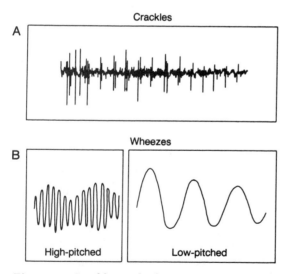

Fig. 15–1. Crackles and wheezes. *A,* Crackles are discontinuous, interrupted explosive sounds with a wide spectrum of frequencies. *B,* Wheezes are continuous sounds that can be high-pitched (composed of multiple frequencies) or low-pitched (composed of fewer frequencies).

MECHANISMS

Crackles

A deflated, excised lung does not inflate smoothly or evenly. Instead, small groups of surface alveoli expand suddenly causing a crackling sound (Fig. 15–1A). Inflation does not produce crackling if the lung is only partially deflated because no alveoli are collapsed. These observations suggest that crackling is due to the sudden equalization of pressure between two areas of the lung containing gas at widely different pressures.

The inspiratory crackles heard while examining a patient result from similar explosive pressure equalization between gas compartments within the lung. The barrier to pressure equalization is an airway that remains closed until its resistance is overcome by the inflating force. Radial traction on airway walls increases during inspiration (see Fig. 6–1). A critical transmural pressure will be reached if these walls are apposed at the beginning of inspiration. The walls will then abruptly separate and rapid equalization between the upstream and downstream pressure occurs. Gas is set in transient oscillation by this brief equalization period and an individual crackle is generated. The critical importance of transmural pressure gradients generating these crackles has been confirmed by simultaneous recording of sound and esophageal pressures. Such experiments show that crackles occur at the same transmural pressure in several consecutive respiratory cycles.[1-5]

Any condition that contributes to the closure of small airways is likely to be associated with *late* inspiratory crackling (Fig. 15–2A). One common contributor is the weight of the overlying lung; its significance can be demonstrated by altering the patient's position. This is sometimes sufficient to expand the basal lung areas to a volume that opens the airways throughout the respiratory cycle, and the crackles are silenced. Other mechanisms that may contribute to airway closure include interstitial edema, diffuse interstitial fibrosis, alveolar filling, and loss of lung volume. Gravity becomes a less important mechanism when these pathologic conditions are sufficiently severe; crackling is then unaffected by changes in posture. Characteristically, these crackles are heard late in the inspiratory cycle, are repetitive with each breath, and are not extinguished by coughing.

Early inspiratory sounds tend to be short, discontinuous, and low pitched.[5-7] Unlike late inspiratory crackles, they are audible at the mouth as well as over the lower lobes, are unaffected by changes in posture, and are often associated with similar sounds in the late phases of exhalation (Fig. 15–2B). These sounds are generated by the passage of gas boluses through intermittently occluded airways. The occluded segment is opened by an explosive equalization of upstream and downstream pressures, and a crackle is generated. These sounds are common in patients with severe congestive heart failure and chronic obstructive pulmonary disorders. Their timing suggests that their source is the lower lobe bronchi or its segmental branches. Fluid in the airway may contribute to crackling because coughing often extinguishes these sounds in severe heart failure. A fold of mucosa, a poorly supported bronchial wall, or mucus in the airways may interrupt air flow in patients with obstructive lung disease. Mucus obstruction seems likely when coughing silences these crackles. Clinical distinctions between early and late crackles provide information about diagnostic categories of lung diseases (Table 15–1).

Crackles found during early, middle, and late inspiration (Fig. 15–2C) may be due to combinations of diseases, such as mild congestive heart failure in patients with chronic obstructive lung disease.

Wheezes

Although these adventitious sounds last only one-half of a second, they are described as continuous because their duration is considerably longer

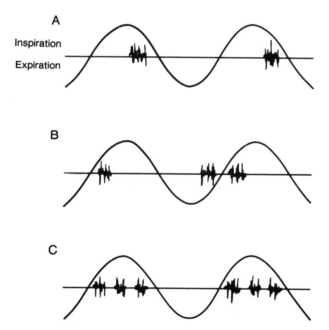

Fig. 15–2. Timing of crackles. A, Late inspiratory crackles. B, Early inspiratory crackles and late expiratory crackles. C, Pan-inspiratory crackles (e.g., found throughout inspiration.)

Table 15-1. Comparisons between early and late inspiratory crackles

Physical findings	Early	Late
Lung zones	Lower	Lower to mid
Gravity dependent		
Dependent	No	Yes
Scanty	Yes	No—profuse
Heard at mouth	Yes	No
Diseases		
Obstructive airway disease	Yes	No
Heart failure	Severe	Mild
Interstitial fibrosis	No	Yes
Pneumonia	No	Yes

than the nearly instantaneous crackle with a duration of only several milliseconds.[1-4] Some authors prefer to subclassify these continuous sounds as rhonchi when they are low pitched and wheezes when they are high pitched. Others use these terms to denote the location at which they are heard, but because these distinctions seem artificial and add no additional information, all continuous sounds (except for stridor, see below) will be termed wheezes in this chapter.

Wheezes are generated by regular vibrations of the airway walls that draw their energy from air flow. Originally, it was thought that wheezes were generated by jets of intraluminal air oscillating the bronchus and therefore creating a musical note. According to this theory, wheezes would be generated by branches in the bronchi or strands of mucus in the airway; pitch was felt to be related to the length of the adjoining bronchus. We now know that such a mechanism is impossible because the low pitch of some wheezes would require a tube several feet in length.

Vibrations are generated by a bronchus in which the opposite walls are almost in contact. The walls vibrate rapidly between the nearly opened and nearly closed positions producing a single musical note. The pitch is low or high depending on the size and compliance of the tissue set into motion and the velocity of air flow.

Wheezing can be present during inspiration and expiration. A narrowed or stenotic bronchus usually produces a single musical note. The wheeze will be audible and constant in pitch throughout the respiratory cycle if the stenosis is rigid. The wheeze may vary in pitch between inspiration and expiration if the stenosis is more flexible. Such wheezes are often characteristic of asthma, but no conclusion can be drawn from the pitch of the wheeze regarding its source. High-pitched wheezing may not originate in small, peripheral airways, but rather may be a sign of expiratory dynamic compression of larger airways.

Polyphonic inspiratory and expiratory wheezes are composed of a variety of unrelated musical notes that start and end simultaneously like a dissonant chord. Compression of the opposite walls of several central bronchi creates a set of self-regulating valves, and the vibrations generated are heard as a cluster of musical notes. Many patients with obstructive airway disease have this form of wheezing, but many healthy subjects can produce a similar sound with a maximal forced expiratory effort. Consequently, polyphonic wheezing is indicative of air flow obstruction only if the expiratory effort is submaximal.

Stridor is a specialized type of wheeze that is more prominent during inspiration. Stridor is commonly found with extrathoracic partial upper airway obstruction. It may also be found with relatively fixed and advanced intra-

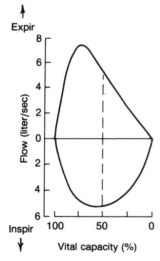

Fig. 15–3. Normal flow volume loop. During expiration, maximal flow occurs at approximately 75% of the vital capacity; during inspiration, maximal flow occurs at 50% of vital capacity. Maximal expiratory flow rate at 50% vital capacity (MEFR 50) should approximately equal maximal inspiratory flow rate (MIFR 50). For example, normal $MEFR_{50}/MIFR_{50} \simeq 1$.

thoracic large airway obstruction. Flow volume loops are helpful in determining the area of obstruction (Figs. 15–3, 15–4).[8]

CRACKLES AND WHEEZES IN SPECIFIC PULMONARY DISEASES

The following table lists certain characteristics of crackles and wheezes in relation to specific pulmonary diseases. Crackles can be classified as early, mid, and late inspiratory or expiratory. A negative (−) sign indicates that crackles are not present. Wheezes are classified as inspiratory, expiratory, or both. Severity of wheezes is as follows: 0 means no wheezes present; 1 is mild—wheezes scattered throughout the chest and noted only after careful auscultation; 2 is moderate—diffuse wheezes are heard immediately on auscultation of the chest; and 3 is severe—diffuse wheezes are heard *without* the aid of a stethoscope.

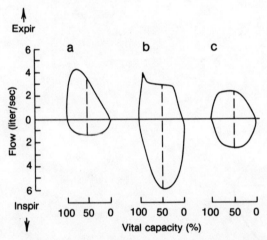

Fig. 15–4. Abnormal flow volume loops. Patients with severe or high grade *extrathoracic* upper airway obstruction (a) may present with stridor. Flow volume loops will display limitation to inspiratory flow (e.g., inspiratory plateau). The $MEFR_{50}/MIFR_{50}$ is >1. Patients with *intrathoracic* airway obstruction (b) display limitation to expiratory flow (e.g., expiratory plateau). The $MEFR_{50}/MIFR_{50}$ < 1. Patients with fixed high-grade *intra-* or *extrathoracic* airway obstruction (c) have plateaus during both inspiration and expiration. The $MEFR_{50}/MIFR_{50} \simeq 1$. A fixed intra- or extrathoracic upper airway obstruction equally decreases maximum inspiratory and expiratory flow rates.

Disease	Crackles	Wheezing	Comments
Obstructive lung disease			
Common			
1. Emphysema	Early inspiratory	Expiratory 0–2	Adventitious sounds are not found in patients with mild to moderate degrees of emphysema. Loss of elastic recoil causes airway narrowing and expiratory wheezing. Early inspiratory crackles are not changed by altering the patient's position and are best heard at the lung bases.
2. Chronic bronchitis	Early inspiratory	Expiratory inspiratory 1–3	Early bibasilar inspiratory crackles and a variety of high- and low-pitched inspiratory and expiratory wheezes are common. The lower pitched wheezes are extinguished by coughing.
3. Asthma	–	Expiratory inspiratory 1–3	Wheezing is characteristic during but not between acute attacks. There is little correlation between the presence and degree of wheezing and the impairment in air flow.
Uncommon			
4. Bronchiectasis	Early inspiratory expiratory	Expiratory inspiratory 1–3	Crackling is similar to that heard in chronic bronchitis, except it tends to be more profuse. Coughing decreases the number of crackles. Wheezing is present in many patients.
5. Cystic fibrosis	Early inspiratory expiratory	Expiratory inspiratory 1–3	Similar to bronchiectasis.
6. Upper airway obstruction	–	Inspiratory expiratory 1–3	Stridor is common in advanced partial obstruction.

Disease	Crackles	Wheezing	Comments

Restrictive lung diseases

Common

7. Interstitial fibrosis	Late inspiratory	0	Late inspiratory crackles are common. Modifiers such as "close to the ear," "cellophane," or "velcro" crackles are used. Such distinctions do not add to our understanding of the underlying disorder or to the physiology of the sound produced. These sounds are usually best heard over the lower lung bases, although with more advanced fibrosis they may be more widespread. Crackles are abolished or altered with changes in position during the early stages of this disease. Coughing does not affect crackles.
8. Sarcoidosis	Late inspiratory	Expiratory 0–1	Crackling is a common finding. Mild obstructive airway disease with expiratory wheezing is occasionally found.
9. Pulmonary edema	Early, mid, and late inspiratory expiratory	Expiratory 1–2	There is poor correlation between these adventitious sounds and the altered hemodynamic measurements in patients with cardiac disease. Some patients have normal breath sounds despite moderate elevations of left ventricular end-diastolic pressure. Late inspiratory crackles are secondary to airway closure caused by interstitial edema. Early inspiratory and late expiratory crackles are found in patients with advanced pulmonary edema. A patient will occasionally also wheeze.

Disease	Crackles	Wheezing	Comments
10. Thoracic cage deformities and abnormalities	Early and late inspiratory	Expiratory 0–1	Lung compression and atelectasis can cause crackles. Bronchial distortion may be responsible for wheezing.
11. Neuromuscular disorders	Late inspiratory	0	The monotonous breathing pattern leads to multiple areas of atelectasis. Late inspiratory crackles are heard with deep breathing.
12. Inhalational or occupational pulmonary diseases	Mid to late inspiratory	Expiratory inspiratory 1–3	A variety of adventitious sounds are found. Patients with byssinosis and industrial asthma wheeze during inspiration and expiration. Patients with asbestosis have crackling characteristics of other forms of interstitial fibrosis. Surprisingly, most patients with coal worker's pneumoconiosis have a normal chest examination.

Uncommon

Disease	Crackles	Wheezing	Comments
13. Hypersensitivity pneumonitis	Late inspiratory	Expiratory inspiratory 1–3	Late inspiratory crackling is common. Patients with bronchospasm experience wheezing.
14. Goodpasture's syndrome	Late inspiratory	0	Crackles are rare.
15. Idiopathic pulmonary hemosiderosis	Late inspiratory	0	Crackles are similar to those found in interstitial fibrosis.
16. Eosinophilic granuloma	Late inspiratory	0	Physical examination is normal except in advanced cases.

Pulmonary vascular disease

Common

Disease	Crackles	Wheezing	Comments
17. Acute pulmonary embolism	Mid to late inspiratory	Expiratory 1–2	Inspiratory crackles are heard when congestive atelectasis is present.

Uncommon

Disease	Crackles	Wheezing	Comments
18. Sickle cell anemia	Late inspiratory	0	Crackles are common because these patients are prone to *in situ* thrombosis, congestive atelectasis, and pneumonias.

Disease	Crackles	Wheezing	Comments
Tumors of the lung, pleura, and mediastinum			
Common			
22. Carcinoma of the lung	Early and late inspiratory	Expiratory inspiratory 1–2	Adventitious sounds are usually not a direct consequence of the neoplasm. Early inspiratory crackles or inspiratory and expiratory wheezes may be a result of the underlying chronic bronchitis or emphysema. Tumor impingement on a major airway may occasionally cause a wheeze. This is characterized by a single musical note not subject to change by respiratory maneuvers such as coughing. Crackles may also be due to postobstructive pneumonias and atelectasis.
23. Metastatic carcinoma of the lung	–	Expiratory 0–1	Metastatic endobronchial carcinoma can partially obstruct airways, producing a wheeze.
25. Bronchial carcinoid	Late inspiratory	Expiratory inspiratory 1–3	Inspiratory and expiratory wheezes are common in the carcinoid syndrome. Adventitious sounds may be due to postobstructive atelectasis.
Infectious diseases of the lung			
Common			
26. Bacterial, mycoplasmal, and rickettsial pneumonias	Late inspiratory	Expiratory 1–2	During the early stages of lobar pneumonia, late inspiratory crackles are common. If the consolidation progresses, the crackles decrease and disappear. Wheezing may be due to mucus in the airways.
27. Viral pneumonias	Late inspiratory	0	
28. Lung abscesses	Mid to late inspiratory	Expiratory 1–2	Lung abscesses may be associated with wheezing when secondary to an endobronchial foreign body or carcinoma.

Disease	Crackles	Wheezing	Comments
29. Tuberculosis	Early inspiratory	Expiratory 1	Adventitious sounds are uncommon. A patient may occasionally have early inspiratory crackles from extensive active disease, pulmonary fibrosis, and bronchiectasis.
Uncommon			
30. Atypical tuberculosis	Early inspiratory	0	
31. *Actinomyces* and *Nocardia*	Mid to late inspiratory	0	
32. Mycoses	Mid to late inspiratory	0	Wheezing and crackling are occasionally heard.
34. Aspiration lung disease	Early, mid, and late inspiratory	Expiratory inspiratory 1–3	The aspiration of irritating solution (e.g., acid gastric content) causes reflex bronchoconstriction and wheezing.
35. Pulmonary alveolar proteinosis	Late inspiratory	0	As the disease progresses and the alveolar filling worsens, crackling may disappear.
36. Wegener's granulomatosis, its variants, and other vasculitides	Mid to late inspiratory	0	

REFERENCES

1. Forgacs P: Lung Sounds. London, Baillière Tindall, 1978
2. Forgacs P: Crackles and wheezes. Lancet 2:203, 1967
3. Forgacs P: The functional basis of pulmonary sounds. Chest 73:399, 1978
4. Murphy RLH, Holford SK: Lung sounds. Basics of Respiratory Diseases 8:1, 1980
5. Nath AR, Capel LH: Inspiratory crackles and mechanical events of breathing. Thorax 29:695, 1974
6. Nath AR, Capel LH: Inspiratory crackles—Early and late. Thorax 29:223, 1974
7. Nath AR, Capel LH: Lung crackles in bronchiectasis. Thorax 35:694, 1980
8. Hyatt RE, Black LF: The flow volume curve. A current perspective. Am Rev Respir Dis 107:191, 1973

16 · CHEST PERCUSSION

FREDERICK L. GLAUSER

Definition
Classification
Mechanisms and Methods
Percussion Notes in Specific Pulmonary Diseases

DEFINITION

Percussion notes are produced by the finger striking the chest directly or indirectly, eliciting a frequency response that is both felt and heard by the examiner. This frequency response depends on the force of percussion, the thickness of the chest wall, and the frequency response of the underlying structures.[1,2]

CLASSIFICATION

The percussion note normally varies in quality in different subjects and over different areas of the chest in the same subject. There are three types of percussion notes:[1]

Normal—the sound generated over the normal lung

Dull—a note of short duration and low intensity without the high-pitched resonance of a normal percussion sound. Normal dullness is found over the liver, the heart, shoulders and scapulae (Figs. 16–1, 16–2). Pathologic dullness is found in patients with pleural effusions, pleural thickening, and parenchymal consolidation.

Tympanitic—sounds with abnormally high-pitched resonance. They are normally found when percussing over a hollow viscus such as the stomach (Fig. 16–1). Pathologic tympany is found in patients with lung hyperinflation (asthma, emphysema), pneumothorax, and large air-containing cysts.

MECHANISMS AND METHODS

There are two methods of percussing: immediate or direct and mediate or indirect. In immediate percussion the chest wall is struck directly with

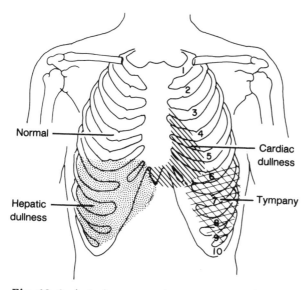

Fig. 16–1. Anterior percussion notes over the normal chest. The boundary between hepatic and cardiac dullness may be difficult to distinguish.

either the palmar aspect of the middle finger or with the tips of all the fingers held together firmly; in mediate (Fig. 16–3), the examiner strikes a pleximeter, which is usually the middle finger of one hand held against the thorax with a plexor. The plexor is the object striking the pleximeter and is usually the middle finger on the other hand. The striking finger causes vibrations of all

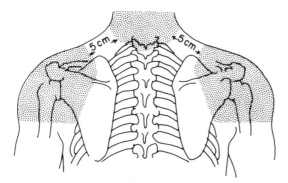

Fig. 16–2. Posterior percussion notes over the normal chest. Dullness is found over both shoulders, the scapulae, and the base of the neck. There is a 5-cm bilateral apical area in which the percussion note is normal.

the surrounding and underlying structures within the areas penetrated by the blow.

The sound waves heard and felt on the chest wall are a composite note produced by the vibrations of the chest wall, underlying tissues (including lungs, liver, and heart), and the pleximeter. This sound is reinforced by the thorax, which acts as a selective resonator and amplifies the lung in the range of 128 cycles per second, the natural frequency of the thorax. The depth of penetration of the vibrating wave into the lung is approximately 5 cm with light percussion. In addition, no lesions less than 2 cm to 3 cm in diameter can be detected.[2]

Descriptions of proper performance for both mediate and immediate percussion can be found in any standard textbook on physical diagnosis. Certain critical points should be stressed, including the following (Fig. 16–3):

1. The middle finger or the pleximeter should be held firmly against the chest wall with all other fingers and the palm raised.
2. The pleximeter should parallel the ribs.
3. The plexor hand should strike short, quick blows—the entire movement being executed from the wrist with the forearm as stationary as possible.
4. A light percussion note should be used because this will enable the examiner to more accurately localize any change in the underlying lung.

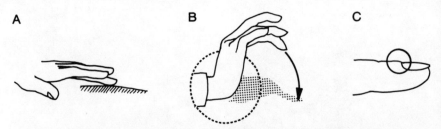

Fig. 16–3. Mediate or indirect percussion. A, The pleximeter (middle finger of the left hand) is held parallel to the ribs with all the other fingers raised from the chest. B, The plexor (right middle finger) strikes short, quick blows, the movement being executed from the wrist with the forearm stationary. C, The plexor strikes the pleximeter at the base of the nail. A light percussion note should be used; sounds on one side of the chest should be compared to sounds on the other side.

5. One side of the thorax should be compared with the opposite side.
6. If at all possible, percussion should be performed with the patient in the sitting position.

When percussing the liver, the examiner should start on the right side of the chest and approach the liver from the apices. The upper liver margin will not be sharply delineated from the normal lung percussion notes. The examiner should measure the total length of the liver, either in inches or centimeters.

Percussion of the heart is imprecise. For adequate evaluation of heart size, radiography is recommended.

Diaphragmatic movement can be determined by percussion (Fig. 16–4). Classically, it was taught that the diaphragm should normally move 5 cm

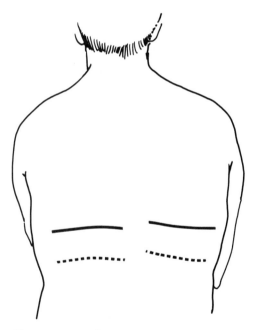

Fig. 16–4. Diaphragmatic movement as determined by percussion. The solid lines represent the upper level of dullness during forced exhalation; the dotted lines represent the lower level of dullness during maximum inhalation. The distance between the two is the maximal diaphragmatic movement, which should be 5 cm to 6 cm.

to 6 cm during maximal inhalation and exhalation. In patients with hyper-inflated lungs (i.e., asthma, emphysema) the excursion is 3 cm to 4 cm.[4,5] Not all authors agree that diaphragmatic movement can be determined accurately using percussion. If evaluation of diaphragmatic excursion is important, inspiratory and expiratory chest radiographs should be obtained.

PERCUSSION NOTES IN SPECIFIC PULMONARY DISEASES

Percussion notes found in specific pulmonary diseases are listed in the following table. The percussion note can be normal, dull, or tympanitic. If the percussion note is dull, this can either be due to pleural effusion (or thickening) or to pulmonary consolidation; if the percussion note is tympanitic, this can be due to a pneumothorax or hyperinflation. If an abnormal percussion note is present, a positive (+) sign will be found in the appropriate column. If neither dullness nor tympany is found, this is indicated by a negative (−) sign (e.g., a normal percussion note is present). A positive/negative sign (±) indicates that the abnormal percussion note occurs infrequently.

Disease	Percussion notes				Comments
	Dullness		Tympany		
	Pleural effusion or thickening	Pulmonary consolidation	Pneumothorax	Hyperinflation	
Obstructive lung disease					
Common					
1. Emphysema	−	−	±	+	Patients with advanced emphysema have a tympanitic percussion note. Because these patients are at an increased risk for pneumothorax, this complication must be ruled out as a cause of tympany.
3. Asthma	−		±	+	Findings are normal between attacks. These patients are at an increased risk of developing spontaneous pneumothorax, and tympany may be due to this complication.
Uncommon					
4. Bronchiectasis	−	+	−	−	Peribronchial fibrosis or a complicating pneumonia can cause a dull percussion note.

Disease	Percussion notes				Comments
	Dullness		Tympany		
	Pleural effusion or thickening	Pulmonary consolidation	Pneumothorax	Hyperinflation	
5. Cystic fibrosis	–	+	–	–	Findings are similar to those in bronchiectasis, although upper lobe dullness may predominate.
Restrictive lung disease					
Common					
9. Pulmonary edema	+	+	–	–	Small bilateral pleural effusions are common in patients with cardiogenic pulmonary edema.
10. Thoracic cage deformities and abnormalities	+	–	–	–	Patients with thoracoplasty have thickened pleurae. Patients with severe kyphoscoliosis may have dullness due to compression of lung tissue.
12. Inhalational or occupational pulmonary disease	+	+	–	–	Dullness is common in patients with silicosis and coal miner's pneumoconiosis who have progressive massive fibrosis. Patients with asbestosis may have pleural thickening.

					Comments
Uncommon					
13. Hypersensitivity pneumonitis	−	+	−	−	In acute hypersensitivity pneumonitis the extensive alveolar filling process produces a dull percussion note.
14. Goodpasture's syndrome	−	+	−	−	
15. Idiopathic pulmonary hemosiderosis	−	+	−	−	
16. Eosinophilic granuloma	−	±	±	−	These patients are at increased risk for spontaneous pneumothorax.
Pulmonary vascular disease					
Common					
17. Acute pulmonary embolism	+	+	−	−	Small pleural effusions are common in patients with pulmonary embolus and infarction. Large emboli or infarctions lead to an alveolar filling process and consolidation.
Uncommon					
18. Sickle cell disease	+	+	−	−	Pleural effusions, pneumonia, and in situ thrombosis can all lead to dullness

[157]

Disease	Percussion notes				Comments
	Dullness		Tympany	Hyper-inflation	
	Pleural effusion or thickening	Pulmonary consoli-dation	Pneumo-thorax		
Tumors of the lung, pleura, and mediastinum					
Common					
22. Carcinoma of the lung	+	+	—	—	Malignant effusions and post-obstructive pneumonias both produce dullness. In most patients with carcinoma there are no abnormal findings.
23. Metastatic carcinoma of the lung	+	—	—	—	Pleural effusions and large parenchymal metastases may cause dullness.
Uncommon					
24. Malignant mesothelioma	+	—	—	—	Pleural effusions and pleural thickening cause dullness.
Infectious diseases of the lung					
Common					
26. Bacterial, mycoplasmal, and rickettsial pneumonias	+	+	—	—	Lobar pneumonias, empyemas, and parapneumonic effusions are associated with dullness.

	1	2	3	4	Comments
27. Viral pneumonias	±	–	–	–	Small pleural effusions are common in these patients.
28. Lung abscesses	+	+	–	–	In a small percentage of patients with large single lung abscesses, the area above an air–fluid level may be tympanitic.
29. Tuberculosis	+	+	–	–	Parenchymal infiltrates and pleural effusions are common.
Uncommon					
30. Atypical tuberculosis	+	+	–	–	
31. Actinomyces and Nocardia	+	+	–	–	Pulmonary parenchymal involvement and pleural effusions are common.
32. Mycoses	+	+	–	–	
Miscellaneous					
33. Aspiration lung disease	+	+	–	–	Aspiration of large amount of fluid may cause alveolar filling with pulmonary consolidation. Secondary infections can lead to parapneumonic effusions or empyemas.
34. Pulmonary alveolar proteinosis	–	–	–	–	
35. Wegener's granulomatosis, its variants, and other vasculitides	+	+	–	–	

REFERENCES

1. Pulmonary terms and symbols: A report in American College of Chest Physicians, American Thoracic Society. Chest 67:683, 1975
2. Forgacs P: Lung sounds. Br J Dis Chest 63, No 1:1–11, 1969
3. Cherniack RM, Cherniack L: Respiration in Health and Disease, pp 3–32; 68–86. Philadelphia, WB Saunders, 1961
4. Fletcher CM: A clinical diagnosis of pulmonary emphysema: An experimental study. Proc R Soc Med 45:577–584, 1952
5. Schneider IC, Anderson A, Jr: Correlation of clinical signs with ventilatory function and obstructive lung disease. Ann Intern Med 62:477–481, 1965

17 · CARDIAC FINDINGS IN LUNG DISEASE

JAMES A. THOMPSON III

FREDERICK L. GLAUSER

DEFINITION

A variety of both acute and chronic lung diseases can affect or alter myocardial structure and function eventuating in cor pulmonale, right ventricular failure, or cardiac arrhythmias.

Cor pulmonale, or pulmonary heart disease, is defined as right ventricular enlargement secondary to acute or chronic pulmonary hypertension. This results from alterations in lung structure or function.[1,2] Acute and chronic pulmonary hypertension cause ventricular dilatation and hypertrophy, respectively. Cor pulmonale can only be diagnosed if both congenital and newly acquired left-sided heart diseases are excluded as the cause of right ventricular enlargement.

Right ventricular failure is defined physiologically as an elevation in right ventricular end-diastolic pressure with a decrease in cardiac output.[3,4] Clinically, right ventricular gallops and heaves, jugular venous distention, an enlarged liver, and peripheral edema are found. Tricuspid insufficiency is occasionally present.

Cardiac arrhythmias are common and include sinus tachycardia, sinus arrhythmias, atrial premature contractions, ventricular ectopic beats, paroxysmal atrial tachycardia, and multifocal atrial tachycardia.[5-7]

MECHANISMS

Normal Right Ventricular and Pulmonary Hemodynamics and Genesis of Heart Sounds

The right ventricle pumps the entire cardiac output (approximately 5 liter/min) through the low-pressure, high-compliance, easily distensible, and recruitable pulmonary vascular bed. In normal subjects at rest and with moderate exercise, the pulmonary artery and right ventricular pressures tend to remain stable, maintaining their normal values of 18–25/6–10 mm Hg and 18–25/0–5 mm Hg, respectively.

The first heart sound (S1) is produced by the closure of the mitral and tricuspid valves at the beginning of ventricular systole. The second heart sound (S2) marks the end of ventricular systole and is associated with closure of the aortic and pulmonic valves. Normally, the aortic valve closes several milliseconds before the pulmonic valve, with this time difference widening during inspiration. Most right-sided cardiac events, whether heart sounds, gallops, murmurs, or ventricular heaves, are accentuated during inspiration as venous return increases.[4]

Physiology and Cardiac Events During the Development of Cor Pulmonale

The cause of the pulmonary arterial hypertension that eventuates in cor pulmonale depends on the specific underlying disease process. Conceptually, it is due to a loss of "effective" units in the pulmonary vascular bed. This loss can be accomplished by some combination of a decrease in lung volume (e.g., interstitial fibrosis), mechanical vascular obstruction (e.g., pulmonary emboli) or pulmonary arterial vasoconstriction with subsequent muscular hyperplasia. Pulmonary arterial vasoconstriction is mediated by some combination of alveolar hypoxia, a low mixed venous oxygen tension, respiratory acidosis, and possibly hypercapnea.[1]

Chronic cor pulmonale and subsequent right ventricular failure is associated with the following events: an elevation in the right ventricular systolic pressure with subsequent hypertrophy of the right ventricular muscle mass as pulmonary artery pressures increase. Right ventricular end-diastolic pressure, volume, and cardiac output are normal at rest and during exercise. Physical examination is normal or reveals a pulmonic second sound equal to or louder than the aortic second sound and a parasternal right ventricular heave. Right ventricular end-diastolic volume increases, preserving resting and exercise cardiac output at the expense of increased myocardial oxygen consumption as pulmonary hypertension progresses. Physical examination may detect a right ventricular gallop that becomes louder during inspiration. Right ventricular end-diastolic pressure and volume increase further as the right ventricle fails. Resting and exercise cardiac output then fall, and jugular venous distention, hepatic engorgement, and peripheral edema are evident.[1]

Jugular Venous Distention

Right atrial pressure can be indirectly estimated by measuring jugular venous distention. The internal jugular veins empty into the superior vena cava, which itself empties into the right atrium. The external jugular joins the subclavian vein, which also empties into the superior vena cava. Elevation of right atrial pressure will be reflected as distention of the external or internal jugular veins. The jugular veins distend when their hydrostatic pressure exceeds atmospheric pressure. This measurement is valid if increased intrathoracic pressure from tachypnea, coughing, laughing, crying, and other Valsalva-like maneuvers are absent. Examination of the external jugular venous system is a less reliable indicator of right atrial pressure and volume status than is evaluation of the internal jugular veins.

Normally, the internal jugular veins partially collapse during inspiration as intrapleural pressure becomes more negative. Failure of this inspiratory collapse to occur may indicate an obstruction to the venous system.

The clinical technique for measuring central venous pressure is simple, reproducible, noninvasive, and requires practice and patience. The observer should search for skin pulsations along the course of the jugular veins while the examination is performed from the anterior or lateral side of the patient (Fig. 17-1). A more distinct wave form will be produced if the opposite jugular vein is occluded with the thumb at the angle of the jaw. The jugular veins are normally distended 2 cm or 3 cm above the sternal angle with the patients in a position 45° from the horizontal. The patient may exhibit venous distention somewhere along the arc from the horizontal to the upright sitting position. Patients should be examined in the sitting, 45°, and supine positions to ascertain the exact height of the jugular venous column. The usual point of reference is the angle of Louis, or where the manubrium and sternum meet with the attachment of the second rib (Fig. 17-2). This angle is approximately

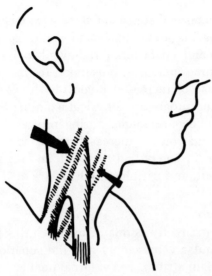

Fig. 17–1. Jugular venous distention. The external jugular vein lies superficial to the sternocleidomastoid muscle; the internal jugular vein lies between the heads of the sternocleidomastoid. Distention of these veins usually indicates increases in right atrial pressure or volume.

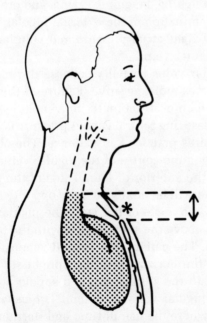

Fig. 17–2. Measurement of jugular venous distention with the patients in the upright position. Horizontal lines are drawn from the angle of Louis (*) and from the highest visible point of jugular venous distention. The distance between these lines (↕) is the jugular venous distention, measured in centimeters.

5 cm H$_2$O above the right atrium in almost all positions. Neck vein height can be estimated or measured by the number of centimeters above or below this point (Fig. 17–2, 17-3).

Persistent elevation of jugular venous pressure is one of the earliest and most reliable signs of right ventricular failure. Analysis of the wave forms may occasionally give additional clues to the underlying disease processes.[6]

CARDIAC ARRHYTHMIAS IN PATIENTS WITH LUNG DISEASE

Patients with chronic obstructive pulmonary disease, acute and chronic respiratory failure from any cause, and pulmonary involvement secondary to a multiorgan system disease (e.g., sarcoidosis, collagen vascular disease) are prone to arrhythmias. In pulmonary diseases in which the heart is

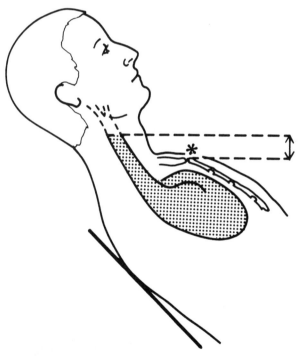

Fig. 17–3. Measurement of jugular venous distention with the patient in the 45-degree position; the same procedure as described in Figure 17-2 is used. Parallel horizontal lines are drawn from the angle of Louis (*) and the highest visible jugular venous distention. The distance between these lines (‡) is the jugular venous distention, measured in centimeters.

not directly affected, the cause of the arrhythmias is multifactorial and includes the effects of hypoxemia, respiratory acidosis and alkalosis, hypocapnea and hypercapnea, elevated pulmonary artery pressures, enlarged and dilated right atrium and ventricles, and drugs such as aminophylline, beta-adrenergic bronchodilators, and diuretics. Whether these arrhythmias contribute to morbidity and mortality is unclear.[6,7]

MISCELLANEOUS EFFECTS OF LUNG DISEASE ON CARDIAC FINDINGS

In patients with marked hyperinflation (e.g., acute asthma and emphysema) heart sounds may be distant and difficult to interpret because of the increased amount of air-containing lung between the examiner and the heart. Heart sounds cannot be heard in the chest, but an epigastric pulsation can be felt and auscultation can be performed in this area, particularly in patients with emphysema. In addition, in patients with diffuse wheezes or crackles, heart sounds may be difficult to interpret during the respiratory cycle.

CARDIAC FINDINGS IN SPECIFIC PULMONARY DISEASES

Cor pulmonale, right ventricular failure, and arrhythmias found in specific pulmonary diseases are listed in the following table. A positive (+) sign indicates that one or more of these conditions is common; a negative (−) sign indicates these conditions do not occur in the specific disease process; and a positive/negative (±) sign means that these conditions occur but are infrequent or uncommon.

Disease	Cor pulmonale and right ventricular failure	Arrhythmias	Comments
Obstructive lung disease			
Common			
1. Emphysema	−	+	Cor pulmonale is precipitated by factors that worsen hypoxemia and hypercapnea. Arrhythmias are common. Distant heart sounds and epigastric cardiac pulsations

Disease	Cor pulmonale and right ventricular failure	Arrhythmias	Comments
			are found in patients with increased anteroposterior chest diameters.
2. Chronic bronchitis	+	+	Patients with chronic hypercapnea and hypoxemia develop cor pulmonale and right ventricular failure. Heart sounds may be difficult to interpret due to the presence of wheezes.
3. Asthma	–	±	Hypoxemia, acute hypocapnea or hypercapnea, acute respiratory alkalosis or acidosis, aminophylline therapy, and other bronchodilator drugs make these patients more susceptible to arrhythmias during acute attacks.
Uncommon			
4. Bronchiectasis	+	±	Cor pulmonale and right ventricular failure are common in patients with diffuse bronchiectasis.
5. Cystic fibrosis	+	±	The findings are similar to patients with bronchiectasis but occur at an earlier age.
6. Upper airway obstruction	±	±	Patients with undiagnosed chronic upper airway obstruction may present with cor pulmonale and right ventricular failure. The initial misdiagnosis is one of intrinsic pulmonary disease. The pulmonary hypertension is caused by the persistent hypoxemia, hypercapnea, and respiratory acidosis. Relief of the upper airway obstruction leads to reversal of hypoxemia and cor pulmonale.

Disease	Cor pulmonale and right ventricular failure	Arrhythmias	Comments
Restrictive lung disease			
Common			
7. Interstitial fibrosis	±	±	Progressive loss of lung volume (vital capacity 50% of predicted), hypoxemia, and hypercapnea cause cor pulmonale in patients with advanced disease.
8. Sarcoidosis	±	±	A small percentage of patients experience progressive pulmonary fibrosis and cor pulmonale. Arrhythmias and sudden death may be due to myocardial sarcoid involvement.
9. Pulmonary edema	±	±	Pulmonary hypertension is common in patients with severe, noncardiogenic pulmonary edema. Acute cor pulmonale and right ventricular failure may be preterminal. Arrhythmias secondary to pulmonary hypertension, blood gas abnormalities, and sepsis are common. Arrhythmias are common because of intrinsic cardiac disease in patients with left ventricular failure.
10. Thoracic cage deformities and abnormalities	±	±	Right ventricular failure may be preterminal.
12. Inhalational or occupational pulmonary diseases	±	±	Cor pulmonale and right ventricular failure are common in patients with progressive pulmonary fibrosis (i.e., silicosis). Arrhythmias are secondary to hypoxemia and pulmonary hypertension.

Disease	Cor pulmonale and right ventricular failure	Arrhythmias	Comments
Uncommon			
13. Hypersensitivity pneumonitis	±	±	Right heart failure secondary to pulmonary hypertension is uncommon, being found in patients with progressive interstitial fibrosis.
Pulmonary vascular diseases			
Common			
17. Acute pulmonary embolism	±	±	Acute cor pulmonale and right ventricular failure may be found in a small percentage of patients with massive pulmonary emboli. Atrial arrhythmias and ventricular fibrillation are common in these patients.
Uncommon			
18. Sickle cell disease	±	±	Chronic cor pulmonale develops in a small percentage of patients.
19. Recurrent pulmonary thromboembolism	+	+	Cor pulmonale, right ventricular failure, and arrhythmias are common.
20. Primary pulmonary hypertension	+	+	Cor pulmonale is common. Most patients die from progressive right heart failure and intractable arrhythmias.
21. Pulmonary veno-occlusive disease	±	+	Pulmonary edema and pulmonary hypertension with eventual right heart failure are common.

Disease	Cor pulmonale and right ventricular failure	Arrhythmias	Comments
Tumors of the lung, pleura, and mediastinum			
Common			
22. Carcinoma of the lung	−	±	Arrhythmias may be due to direct extension of the tumor into the pericardium and myocardium.
Uncommon			
24. Malignant mesothelioma	−	+	Malignant mesothelioma can extend directly into the pericardium and myocardium.
Infectious disease of the lung			
Common			
26. Bacterial, mycoplasmal, or rickettsial pneumonias	−	+	Pneumonias adjacent to the heart may be associated with atrial fibrillation and atrial arrhythmias. Hypoxemia and acid–base inbalances may also contribute to these abnormalities.
29. Tuberculosis	−	+	Arrhythmias in these patients may be due to tuberculous pericarditis and hypoxemia.
Miscellaneous			
38. Sleep apnea, central hypoventilation syndromes	+	+	Hypoxemia, chronic hypercapnea, and respiratory acidosis lead to pulmonary hypertension and cor pulmonale. Right ventricular failure is common. Sleep-induced arrhythmias include sinus bradycardia and arrests, premature atrial contractions, and occasionally ventricular tachycardia and fibrillation.

REFERENCES

1. Fishman AP: Chronic cor pulmonale. In Lung Diseases: State of the Art, 1976–1977, pp. 355–375. New York, American Lung Association, 1978
2. Ferrer MI: Cor pulmonale (pulmonary heart disease): Present day status. Am Heart J 89:657, 1975
3. Harvey RM, Ferrer MI, Richards DW, Jr. et al: The influence of chronic pulmonary disease on the heart and circulation. Am J Med 10:719–738, 1951
4. Fishman AP: Dynamics of the pulmonary circulation. In Hamilton WF, Dowell P (eds): Handbook of Physiology, Section II, Vol. 2. Washington, DC, American Physiological Society, 1963
5. Senior RN, Lefrak SS, Kleiger RE: The heart in chronic obstructive pulmonary disease. Arrhythmias. Chest 75:1–2, 1979
6. Hudson LD, Kurt TL, Petty TL et al: Arrhythmias associated with acute respiratory failure in chronic airway obstruction. Chest 63:661–665, 1973
7. Kleiger RE, Senior RM: Long term electrocardiographic monitoring of ambulatory patients with chronic airway obstruction. Chest 65:483–487, 1974

18 · CLUBBING AND HYPERTROPHIC OSTEOARTHROPATHY

BARBARA PHILLIPS

CLUBBING

Definition

Clubbing refers to painless, uniform enlargement of the terminal segment of a finger or toe. Clubbing is occasionally referred to as Hippocratic fingers because it was first described by Hippocrates in the fifth century BC. Other synonyms include watch-glass nails, parrot-beak nails, drumstick fingers, and essential dactylomegaly.

Early or minimal clubbing is often quite difficult to recognize, and even experienced clinicians are apt to disagree whether a given digit is clubbed (Fig. 18–1). The following are criteria for clubbing:

1. A change in the angle between the nail and the proximal skin to 180° or more.
2. Increased hyponychial angle
3. Ratio of distal phalangeal depth (DPD) to interphalangeal depth (IPD) greater than 1
4. Increased bulk of the terminal digital tuft

172

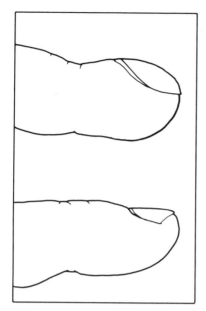

Fig. 18–1. Far advanced clubbing compared to normal. In the upper figure there is obvious loss of angle between the nail and nailbed compared to the normal nail. The angle is greater than 200° in this example.

5. Sponginess of the nail bed
6. Increased nail curvature

Of the criteria listed, loss of the angle between the nail and nail bed (the normal angle is 160° to 165° for fingers and 175° for thumbs) is the earliest, most reliable, and most important sign (Fig. 18–1).[1,2] Clubbing is present if the hyponychial angle (as measured on a tracing of a finger) that normally averages 187°, is increased to 209° (Fig. 18–2).[3]

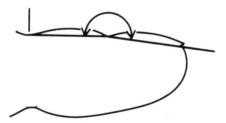

Fig. 18–2. Determination of hyponychial angle. In this illustration, the hyponychial angle is less than 180°, and clubbing is not present. If the hyponychial angle exceeds 209°, clubbing is present.

Another objective method of confirming clubbing is to measure the depth of the index finger at the base of the nail (DPD) and divide by the depth at the interphalangeal joint (IPD) (Fig. 18–3). A DPD/IPD ratio greater than 1 is an objective indication of clubbing.[4] Less reliable signs include sponginess of the nail bed and an increase in the bulk of the terminal tuft, which can be seen in other conditions such as acromegaly and chronic paronychia. Because of the great variability in the saggittal curvature of normal nails, an exaggerated curvature may be mistaken for clubbing.

Mechanisms

The mechanisms responsible for clubbing remain unclear, but several hypotheses have been advanced:

Circulating Vasodilators—A variety of circulating vasodilators (e.g., carbonic acid, ferritin, prostaglandins, bradykinins, adenine nucleotides, and 5-hydroxytryptamine) are hypothesized to be released by normal tissues and escape degradation by the lung through left to right shunts.

Tissue Hypoxia—Tissue hypoxia induces clubbing in patients with congenital cyanotic heart disease by some unknown direct effect.

Neural Mechanisms—A vagal mechanism is hypothesized to play a role in the genesis of clubbing. There is little evidence to support this concept.

Genetic Factors—Hereditary clubbing is common. Investigators have extrapolated from this data and postulated that patients who develop clubbing later in life may have a genetic predisposition.

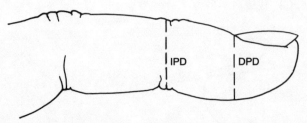

Fig. 18–3. DPD/IPD ratio. The depth of the index finger at the base of the nail (DPD) is divided by the depth of the interpharyngeal joint (IPD) to determine whether clubbing is present. A ratio greater than 1 is an objective indicator of clubbing.

Incidence and Characteristics

Clubbing is reported to occur in 2% to 48% of hospitalized patients. This variability is probably due to the improper application of the diagnostic criteria discussed above and confusion of this entity with hypertrophic osteoarthropathy (HOA). The following are nonpulmonary causes of clubbing:

Cardiac—congenital cyanotic heart disease, subacute bacterial endocarditis (i.e., aortic or mitral involvement most common), and chronic congestive heart failure (particularly due to mitral stenosis)

Hepatic—hypertrophic biliary cirrhosis, toxic cirrhosis, obstructive cirrhosis, portal cirrhosis (rare), and cirrhosis secondary to hemochromatosis (very rare)

Gastrointestinal—ulcerative colitis, chronic bacillary or amebic dysentary, Crohn's disease, colonic carcinoma, multiple colonic polyposis, sprue and celiac sprue, intestinal ascariasis, pyloric obstruction (uncommon)

Endocrine—pregnancy (clubbing may reverse with delivery), myxedema, cretinism, and postthyroidectomy for Graves' disease

Miscellaneous—purpura rheumatica, chronic cystopyelitis, syringomyelia, chronic nephritis, polycythemia rubra vera, and recurrent subluxation of the shoulder (rare)

Clubbing is more common in men than in women, is usually symmetrical, and often involves the toes as well as the fingers. Unilateral clubbing may be found in association with localized aneurysmal dilatations of the aortic arch or one of its branches and with upper extremity arterial venous malformations. Unidigital, nasal, ear, eyelid, and malar clubbing have all been described.[11]

Many patients with acquired clubbing are unaware of the changes in their fingers, but may notice that the nails and cuticle of the clubbed digits grow faster than normal. This results in frequent nail clipping and an increased incidence of acute and chronic paronychia. On examination, the skin of the affected phalanx is often flushed, and the nail bed may be tightly stretched, thin, and shiny. Dorsiflexion of the distal phalanx may develop in patients with chronic clubbing.

Once present, clubbing tends to persist even when the underlying disease process is appropriately treated; however, clubbing may resolve when associated with the hypertrophic osteoarthropathy syndrome. Treatment of hypothyroidism with thyroid replacement and ligation of an associated aneurysm may relieve clubbing.

Histology and Physiology of Clubbed Fingers

Increased deposition of vascular connective tissue is primarily responsible for the increase in size of the soft tissues.[6] Clubbing becomes irreversible once collagen is laid down. There is an increase in blood flow to the affected digits in acquired versus hereditary clubbing. Numerous dermal arterial venous anastomoses in the digital tips, nail beds, palms, soles, lips, cheeks, ears, and forehead have been found, and increased blood flow traverses these anastomoses.[7] The absence of clubbing in patients with anemia and thyrotoxicosis associated with increased dermal blood flow, may be explained by the low number of arterial venous anastomoses present.

HYPERTROPHIC OSTEOARTHROPATHY

Definition and Mechanisms

Hypertrophic osteoarthropathy (HOA) consists of nonpitting swelling, warmth, and tenderness of the tissues covering the ends of long bones; radiographic appearance of periosteal new bone formation (periostitis); arthralgias; and clubbing (not invariably present). Nonpulmonary causes are as follows:

1. Any condition that causes clubbing can also be associated with HOA. The exception is hepatic cirrhosis, in which HOA is reportable.
2. Chronic methemoglobinemia
3. Chronic sulfhemoglobinemia
4. Gynecomastia with increased estrogen secretion
5. Infected abdominal aortic prosthesis
6. Amebiasis
7. Ulcerative colitis
8. Sprue
9. Ascariasis
10. Chronic mountain sickness
11. Pregnancy

As with clubbing, the mechanisms responsible for HOA remain unclear, but several have been postulated.

Theories and Mechanisms Regarding the Etiology of HOA

Circulating vasodilators—Because HOA rarely occurs in association with right-to-left shunting, a chemical substance produced by hypoxic tissues is unlikely to be the causative agent.

Tissue hypoxia—Hypoxia is an unlikely mediator because HOA is rare in cyanotic states.

Immunological mechanisms—Because HOA may be associated with fevers, elevated erythrocyte sedimentation rates, and polyarteritis nodosa and responds to steroid administration, an inflammatory immunologic basis has been postulated.

Hormonal causes—Similarities between acromegaly and HOA have prompted investigators to hypothesize an endocrinological basis for the osteoarthropathy, but there is little evidence to support this theory.

Genetic factors—Pachydermoperiostitis, the hereditary form of HOA, is inherited as a recessive, dominant or sex-linked trait. In contrast to HOA, limb blood flow is normal, so they are not likely to have similar etiologies.

Neural mechanisms—There are several observations that point to a neurogenic basis as a cause for the HOA: vagotomy may relieve the signs and symptoms of HOA whereas this procedure has little effect on clubbing; severing of the lung pedicle or anesthetic block of the cervical vagus nerve reduces blood flow to the HOA-effected limb; mediastinal and vagal involvement secondary to aortic aneurysms and Hodgkin's disease is associated with a high incidence of HOA; the majority of diseases associated with HOA affect the viscera supplied by the ninth and tenth cervical nerves; and pleural efferent vagal fibers have been implicated in the pathogenesis of HOA because peripheral bronchial carcinomas, pleural metastasis, and pleural fibromas are associated with osteoarthropathy whereas central bronchogenic carcinomas are not.

Conversion from simple clubbing to HOA and intermediate forms sometimes occurs, as in clubbing associated with periostitis. Clubbing is more frequent than HOA and implies a more benign prognosis. Clubbing is frequently hereditary or associated with benign disease, whereas 90% of HOA cases are associated with intrathoracic neoplasms.[5]

Incidence and Characteristics

HOA is found in 3% to 5% of all lung cancers but in 60% of fibrous tumors of the pleura. The striking male predominance probably reflects the high incidence of lung cancer in men. HOA may appear 6 months to 20 years after the onset of the underlying disease and is often asymptomatic during the initial stages.[1]

Joint pain secondary to HOA may be the first manifestation of bronchogenic carcinoma. Soft tissue swelling predominates in the distal portions of the extremities, in contrast to acromegaly.[5] The arthritis of HOA resembles a subacute inflammatory rheumatic condition with varying degrees of pain and local swelling unresponsive to standard therapy. The pain is aggravated by cold or movement and may intensify or ameliorate during the menses. Facial features become slightly more prominent in one third of patients.

Patients with HOA may develop an awkward gait and clumsiness of the fingers because of the increased size and weight of the long bones.[1] Associated peripheral neurovascular disorders such as increased local sweating, paresthesias, and chronic erythema may be noted.

The most commonly affected joints are the ankles (88%), wrists (82.5%), and knees (75%), with the elbows, shoulders and fingers involved less often. Small effusions and reduced range of motion may occur in affected joints, and ankylosis may develop in chronic cases.

The bone change is a bilateral proliferating periostitis, involving the radius, fibula, ulna, tibia, phalanges, femor, metacarpals, metatarsals, humerus, and pelvis. The skull and other bones are generally unaffected. Radiologically, the periostitis appears either as a regular sheath of variable length along the diaphysis or as an irregularly ridged layer. Technetium pyrophosphate bone scans may be helpful in establishing the diagnosis when the periostitis is difficult to detect radiologically because they are more sensitive in detecting new bone formation than are standard radiographs.[8]

In general, any treatment or procedure that improves the underlying condition may cause immediate symptom relief and regression of the signs of HOA.[9] The arthralgias may take hours, the edema weeks, and the clubbing months to resolve. The bony changes reverse more slowly and incompletely.

Complete resolution of symptoms and of some of the signs of HOA have been noted after spontaneous or surgical drainage of an empyema or lung abscesses, cure of pneumonias, surgical or radiation treatment of bronchiectasis, collapse therapy for tuberculosis, treatment of pulmonary syphilis, severing of the vagus nerve, removal or radiation of primary lung lesions, following exploratory thoracotomy, and postpartum.[1,10,11] Improvement has also been seen after successful medical or surgical treatment of amebiasis, ulcerative colitis, sprue, and ascariasis and following descent to sea level in patients with chronic mountain sickness.

Histology and Physiology of Hypertrophic Osteoarthropathy

HOA is characterized by edema, new bone formation, and an increase in limb blood flow as well as periostial arteriovenous anastomoses through which much of the increased blood flow passes. In pachydermoperiostosis, just as in congenital clubbing, blood flow is normal and the arterioles are narrowed.

Differential Diagnosis

The differential diagnosis of HOA includes rheumatoid arthritis, osteoarthritis, localized chronic edema, thyroid acropachy, elephantiasis, and acromegaly. The synovial fluid in HOA is usually clear, with decreased viscosity, a low protein concentration, and fewer than 500 leukocytes/mm^3, predominantly lymphocytes and mononuclear cells. The noninflammatory nature of the fluid is inconsistent with a diagnosis of rheumatoid arthritis. The radiologic findings in HOA do not mimic those of osteoarthritis. The bone pain, lack of pitting edema and joint effusions, and frequent lack of obvious etiology should dissuade the physician from making a diagnosis of chronic edema, elephantiasis, or thyroid acropachy. As in acromegaly, suppression of growth hormone secretion during glucose tolerance testing may be impaired in HOA; however, patients with acromegaly do not have periostitis. The finding of periosteal new bone formation in a patient without bone or joint pain, ankle edema, joint stiffness, or synovial effusions suggests a diagnosis of syphilis, scurvy, or an overdose of fluoride, strontium, or vitamin A or D.

Pachydermoperiostosis is a rare syndrome and resembles HOA except that the joint and bone pains are usually less severe, and there is no associated disease. It should not be confused with hereditary or primary clubbing, which does not have the bony changes found in HOA. Pachydermoperiostosis is often familial and may first be noticed at the time of puberty. It is associated with thickening and seborrheic changes of the skin of the forehead, nose, and scalp. The condition is termed cuticus verticus gyrata when the skin changes are prominent.

CLUBBING AND HYPERTROPHIC OSTEOARTHROPATHY IN SPECIFIC PULMONARY DISEASES

The presence of clubbing and hypertrophic osteoarthropathy in specific pulmonary diseases is listed in the following table. A positive (+) sign means that either clubbing or hypertrophic osteoarthropathy occurs relatively frequently in a specific disease; a negative (−) sign means that clubbing or hypertrophic osteoarthropathy is rare or *does not* occur in a specific disease.

Disease	Club-bing	Hypertrophic osteo-arthropathy	Comments
Obstructive lung disease			
Common			
2. Chronic bronchitis	+	−	Clubbing is rare and unrelated to the severity of the disease or the degree of hypoxemia.
Uncommon			
4. Bronchiectasis	+	−	Clubbing is common and can be quite striking.
5. Cystic fibrosis	+	−	There is evidence that the severity of finger clubbing is related to the degree of pulmonary involvement.
Restrictive lung disease			
Common			
7. Interstitial fibrosis	+	−	Clubbing is almost universally present in chronic, advanced cases.
10. Thoracic cage deformities and abnormalities	+	−	There is a high incidence of clubbing in patients with thoracic cage deformities from chronic empyemas.
Tumors of the lung, pleura, and mediastinum			
Common			
22. Carcinoma of the lung	+	+	Clubbing is common and may regress completely if the underlying tumor is treated appropriately. Bronchogenic carcinoma is the most common cause of HOA. Squamous cell carcinoma is the most common histologic type, followed by adenocarcinoma. Large cell, undifferentiated, and alveolar cell carcinomas are rarely associated with HOA, which occurs in approximately 5% of small cell carcinomas. The appearance of osteoarthropathy coincides with the onset of pulmonary symptoms

Disease	Club-bing	Hypertrophic osteo-arthropathy	Comments
			in about one third of cases; it precedes the onset of pulmonary symptoms and is the only manifestation of lung cancer in another one third of bronchogenic carcinoma cases. Osteoarthropathy occurs with increased frequency in patients with larger tumors, but despite this relationship, osteoarthropathy has no prognostic implication.
23. Metastatic carcinoma of the lung	+	+	Any tumor that metastasizes to the lung parenchyma or pleura may be associated with clubbing. Metastatic osteogenic sarcoma is one of the few causes of childhood clubbing. The incidence of HOA with metastatic tumors is lower than with primary lung tumors. Tumors most commonly associated with osteoarthropathy include carcinoma of the breast, adrenal glands, pharynx, salivary glands, or bones. HOA associated with metastases carries a grave prognosis.
Uncommon			
24. Malignant mesothelioma	+	+	These tumors account for 10% of all cases of HOA.
Infectious diseases of the lung			
Common			
26. Bacterial, mycoplasmal, and rickettsial pneumonias	−	−	Clubbing has rarely been reported in acute lobar pneumonias. Chronic empyema secondary to pneumonias was once the most common cause of clubbing; however, this entity is now rare with modern medical treatment. The incidence of clubbing has therefore decreased.

Disease	Clubbing	Hypertrophic osteoarthropathy	Comments
28. Lung abscesses	+	−	Clubbing often appears early. There is no relationship between the chronicity or severity of the underlying process and the degree of clubbing. Clubbing may be a premonitory sign of abscess formation. Resolution of lung abscesses or empyemas may reverse the clubbing.
29. Tuberculosis	+	−	Clubbing occurs primarily in patients with chronic pulmonary tuberculosis associated with fibrosis, cavitation, or bronchiectasis. Clubbing is associated with a higher incidence of hemoptysis, weight loss, large cavities, and increased mortality.
Uncommon			
30. Atypical tuberculosis	+	−	Clubbing is usually associated with the underlying cystic disease or bronchiectasis.

REFERENCES

1. Mendlowitz M: Clubbing and hypertrophic osteoarthropathy. Medicine 21:269–306, 1942
2. Loribond JL: Diagnosis of clubbed fingers. Lancet 1:363, 1938
3. Regan GM, Tagg B, Thompson ML: Subjective and objective measurement of finger clubbing. Lancet 1:530, 1967
4. Sly RM: Objective assessment for digital clubbing in caucasian, negro, and oriental subjects. Chest 64:687, 1973
5. Coury C: Hippocratic fingers and hypertrophic osteoarthropathy. Br J Dis Chest 54:202, 1960
6. Shneerson JM: Digital clubbing and hypertrophic osteoarthropathy: The underlying mechanisms. Br J Dis Chest 75:113, 1981
7. Racoceanean SN: Digital capillary blood flow in clubbing. ^{85}Kr studies in hereditary and acquired cases. Ann Intern Med 75:933, 1971
8. Lockich JJ: Pulmonary osteoarthropathy. Association with mesenchymal tumors metastoses to the lungs. JAMA 238:37, 1977
9. Rao GM, Guruprakash GH, Poulose K et al: Improvement in hypertrophic pulmonary osteoarthropathy after radiotherapy to metastasis. AJR 133:944, 1979
10. Huckstep RL, Bodkin PE: Vagotomy in hypertrophic pulmonary osteoarthropathy associated with bronchial carcinoma. Lancet 2:343, 1958
11. Borden EC, Holling HE: Hypertrophic osteoarthropathy and pregnancy. Ann Intern Med 71:577, 1969

19 · ASTERIXIS

SCOTT K. RADOW

DEFINITION

Asterixis is a unique neurologic syndrome associated with a variety of disease entities. The name is derived from the Greek: "a" (privation) and "sterixis" (maintenance of posture). Common synonyms include *liver flap* and *flapping tremor*.

MECHANISMS AND DESCRIPTION

Active dorsiflexion of the wrist with the arms outstretched and pronated elicits asterixis in susceptible patients. Passive wrist dorsiflexion is less sensitive and reliable in producing this sign. A characteristic tremor consisting of anteroposterior oscillation of the fingers, tiny random finger movements, and a rotary wrist motion develops following a latent period of 2 to 30 seconds. Asterixis occurs on a background of increasing tremor amplitude and encompasses two major components: a sudden rapid forward hand jerk is followed by an eqally rapid and sudden withdrawal movement that returns the hand to its original dorsiflexed position (Fig. 19–1). These movements are usually repeated two or three times in quick succession. The tremor and asterixis cease briefly, and then an irregular, recurrent sequence is established.[1,2]

Asterixis is usually bilateral. The hands move with similar but asynchronous rates, and the movements are involuntary. Although the standard method of testing for asterixis is to dorsiflex the wrist, virtually any other muscle group that undergoes sustained active contraction can be used. These muscle groups include those that dorsiflex the ankle, knee, and the hip. Protrusion of the tongue, retraction of the mouth corners, and hand grasping may also elicit asterixis.[1,2]

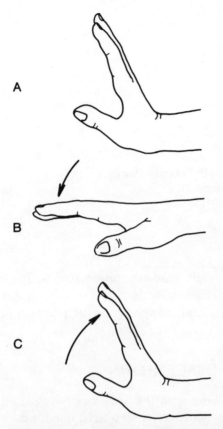

Fig. 19–1. Sequence of hand movement during asterixis. A, The wrist is actively dorsiflexed and the arm outstretched. B, Following a latent period of 2 to 30 seconds, there is a sudden rapid forward hand jerk followed by (C) a rapid, sudden withdrawal movement returning the hand to the original dorsiflexed position.

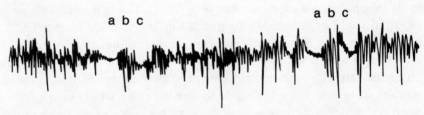

Fig. 19–2. Schematic electromyogram from a patient with asterixis. First period of electrical silence (a) corresponds to the rapid forward hand movement. High voltage burst of electrical activity (b) corresponds to the braking in forward movement of the hand and the onset of active withdrawal. Second period of electrical silence (c) corresponds to the braking and stoppage of the withdrawal motion of the hand.

Asterixis is associated with unique changes in electromyographic (EMG) recordings, regardless of etiology. The EMG is normal with the patient at rest, with passive hand movement, and during phasic voluntary movement. Two to thirty seconds after initiation of a sustained tonic contraction, the recording becomes abnormal (Fig. 19–2). A 50-msec to 100-msec electrically silent period is followed 20 msec to 200 msec later by the forward hand jerk. A burst of high-voltage electrical activity follows, which correlates with the braking of the forward hand motion and the onset of active withdrawal. A second electrically silent period corresponds to the braking and stoppage of the withdrawal movement. The EMG recording then returns to normal until the sequence repeats itself.[3,4]

PATHOPHYSIOLOGY

The underlying neuropathophysiology associated with asterixis remains unclear. Asterixis is most commonly observed in metabolic encephalopathies of diverse etiology, including hypercapnea (chronic pulmonary insufficiency), uremia (chronic renal failure), toxic nitrogenous compounds (hepatic insufficiency), and varied drug intoxications (phenobarbital, etc.). The only element common to these disorders is an altered mental status characterized by decreased consciousness, disorientation, and disordered cerebration. This link is not universal because a small number of patients with normal mentation experience asterixis.[5-9]

Sensory function is typically normal, and focal neurologic deficits of any kind are rare. The electroencephalographic (EEG) pattern is characteristic of a metabolic encephalopathy displaying diffuse, high-voltage slow waves. No unique EEG abnormality is seen even during periods of EMG electrical silence. False neurotransmitters have been postulated to play a role in asterixis, but no specific chemical agent or site of abnormal neurotransmission has been identified. Other possible pathogenetic mechanisms include a primary lapse of cortical output, an inhibitory cortical output to lower motor neurons (LMN), or decreased excitability of the LMN pool with normal cortical output.

Focal lesions in the midbrain, thalamus, and internal capsule have been associated with contralateral asterixis in patients without other neurologic or metabolic derangements.[10-14] Damaged areas include the mesencephalic reticular formation (MRF), cerebellar afferents and efferents, and the basal ganglia. The MRF is responsible for the arousal of higher CNS centers by incoming sensory stimuli; this sensory input is necessary for position maintenance with its loss resulting in a lapse of CNS output to LMNs. The basal ganglia and cerebellum are responsible for gross and fine tuning of position maintenance, respectively. Functional deficits in these regions could also result in a lapse of CNS output to the LMNs.

DIFFERENTIAL DIAGNOSIS

Metabolic encephalopathies are the most common causes of asterixis. Asterixis is an expected finding in severe hepatic and uremic renal failure and is not uncommon in patients with chronic hypercapneic pulmonary disease and in a variety of drug intoxications such as anticonvulsant overdose.[5-9] A 20% incidence during recovery from anesthesia has been reported, although no specific agents have been incriminated.

I. Common
   A. Metabolic encephalopathies
      1. Chronic lung disease with hypercapnea
      2. Hepatic insufficiency
      3. Renal failure with uremia
      4. Drug intoxications (phenytoin, carbamazepine, sodium valproate, bromide, lithium, glutethimide)
   B. Recovery from anesthesia
II. Uncommon
   A. Focal central nervous system deficits
      1. Mesencephalon
      2. Basal ganglia
      3. Internal capsule
   B. Miscellaneous
      1. Hypokalemia
      2. Hypomagnesemia
      3. Congestive heart failure
      4. Malabsorption syndromes
      5. Syndrome of inappropriate ADH secretion
      6. Metrizamide myelography
      7. Hyperparathyroidism with hypercalcemia

CHARACTERISTICS OF PATIENTS WITH PULMONARY DISEASES ASSOCIATED WITH ASTERIXIS

Asterixis occurs in patients with acute decompensation of an underlying chronic pulmonary condition. The majority have obstructive airway disease, although a significant minority have severe advanced restrictive disease. Hypercapnea with $PaCO_2$ varying from 44 torr to 105 torr in the small number of patients with recorded arterial blood gas values is common. Asterixis generally disappears as hypercapnea resolves; however, this is not a universal finding because asterixis worsens in some patients as their Pa_{CO_2} improves. Arterial pH values vary from 7.22 to 7.49. Arterial oxygen desaturation is found in most but not all patients. The relative contributions of pH and oxygen desaturation to the development of asterixis in hypercapneic patients is unknown.[6-8]

Several associated disturbances are found in hypercapneic patients with asterixis, including altered mental status with lethargy, confusion, and disorientation; right ventricular failure; left ventricular failure in approximately one third of the patients; primary metabolic alkalosis secondary to diuretic therapy; and polycythemia in approximately 15% of the patients. Liver and renal function studies are usually normal.

In summary, the only recognized common precipitant for the development of asterixis is an elevated Pa_{CO_2} in a patient with acute decompensation of chronic pulmonary disease. The presence of altered mental status, metabolic alkalosis, and right or left ventricular failure may be contributory. The significance of hypoxemia and altered acid–base states is unknown.

ASTERIXIS IN SPECIFIC PULMONARY DISEASES

In contrast to Chapters 1 through 18, a detailed listing of the specific pulmonary diseases associated with asterixis will not be found in this chapter. Instead, the diseases in which asterixis is found are presented in outline form.

Asterixis in Specific Pulmonary Diseases

Obstructive Lung Diseases
    Emphysema
    Bronchitis
    Asthma (severe)

    Bronchiectasis
    Cystic fibrosis
    Upper airway obstruction
Restrictive Lung Disease
    Interstitial fibrosis
    Sarcoidosis (advanced)
    Thoracic cage deformities and abnormalities (particularly kyphoscoliosis and thoracoplasty)
    Inhalational or occupational pulmonary disease (advanced)

Hypersensitivity pneumonitis (chronic, advanced)
Idiopathic pulmonary hemosiderosis
Tumors of the Lung, Pleura, and Mediastinum
Carcinoma of the lung (with post-obstructive infection)
Infectious Diseases of the Lung
Tuberculosis (advanced)
Miscellaneous
Sleep apnea and central hypoventilation syndromes

REFERENCES

1. Leavitt S, Tyler HR: Studies in asterixis. Arch Neurol 10:360–368, 1964
2. Tyler HR, Leavitt S: Asterixis. J Chronic Dis 18:409–411, 1965
3. Shahani BT, Young RR: Asterixis—A disorder of the neural mechanisms underlying sustained muscle contraction. In Shahani M (ed): The Motor System: Neurophysiology and Muscle Mechanisms. Amsterdam, Elsevier, 1976
4. Adams RD, Foley JM: The disorder of movement in the more common varieties of liver disease. Electroencephalogr Clin Neurophysiol (Suppl) 3:51, 1953
5. Adams RD, Foley JM: The neurological change in the more common types of severe liver disease. Trans Am Neurol Assoc 74:217–219, 1949
6. Westlake EK, Simpson T, Kaye M: Carbon dioxide narcosis in emphysema. Q J Med 24:155–173, 1955
7. Austen FK, Carmichael MW, Adams RD: Neurological manifestations of chronic pulmonary insufficiency. N Engl J Med 257:579–590, 1957
8. Conn HO: Asterixis: Its occurrence in chronic pulmonary disease with a commentary on its general mechanism. N Engl J Med 259:564–569, 1958
9. Conn HO: Asterixis in nonhepatic disorders. Am J Med 29:647–661, 1960
10. Young RR, Shahani BT, Kjellberg RJ: Unilateral asterixis produced by a discrete CNS lesion. Trans Am Neurol Assoc 101:306–307, 1976
11. Tarsy D, Lieberman B, Chirico-Post P et al: Unilateral asterixis associated with a mesencephalic syndrome. Arch Neurol 34:446–447, 1977
12. Dril V, Sharpe JA, Ashby P: Midbrain asterixis. Ann Neurol 6:362–364, 1979
13. Degos JD, Vevvoust J, Bouchareine A et al: Asterixis in focal brain lesions. Arch Neurol 36:705–707, 1979
14. Donat JR: Unilateral asterixis due to thalamic hemorrhage. Neurology 30:83–84, 1980

20 · CYANOSIS

J. EUGENE MILLEN

DEFINITION

Cyanosis is a bluish discoloration of the skin and mucous membranes caused by excessive concentrations of reduced hemoglobin in the subpapillary venous plexus. The amount of reduced hemoglobin depends on the hemoglobin concentration and oxygen saturation, the Po_2 in the arterial and venous blood, and the cardiac output or some combination of these factors.

Cyanosis is discernible when 5 gm/dl or more of reduced hemoglobin or 6.95 vol% or more of unoxygenated hemoglobin is present in capillary blood. Observation of the skin, nail beds, or mucous membranes for cyanosis provides information about the color of the blood at the midcapillary level. This color depends on midcapillary oxygen concentration or content defined as the mean of the arterial and venous values.[1-3]

CLASSIFICATION

Peripheral cyanosis. Arterial oxygen desaturation does *not* exist because the hemoglobin oxygen saturation is greater than 80% to 85%; however, red blood cells lose excessive oxygen to the tissues due to prolonged transit time through the peripheral capillaries. This decreases venous and midcapillary oxygen contents.[4]

Central cyanosis. Arterial oxygen desaturation *does* exist because the hemoglobin oxygen saturation is less than 80% to 85%. This is usually due to a low atmospheric oxygen content such as occurs at high altitude, with pulmonary dysfunction, or with intracardiac shunts.[5]

Combined forms of cyanosis. Both central and peripheral oxygen desaturation are present simultaneously. A common clinical example is observed in patients with myocardial infarctions who have pulmonary edema. This leads to moderate arterial oxygen desaturation and decreased cardiac output causing excess peripheral extraction of oxygen from the blood.

MECHANISMS

The arterial and venous oxygen contents (CaO_2 and CvO_2, respectively) are subtracted from fully saturated hemoglobin to quantitate the total amount of reduced or unoxygenated hemoglobin in the capillaries.

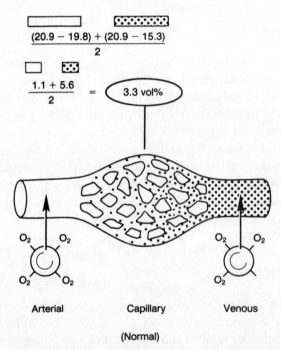

$$\frac{(20.9 - 19.8) + (20.9 - 15.3)}{2}$$

$$\frac{1.1 + 5.6}{2} = \boxed{3.3 \text{ vol\%}}$$

Arterial   Capillary   Venous

(Normal)

Fig. 20–1. Normal patient. The hemoglobin concentration, CaO_2, and CvO_2, and cardiac output are normal. The arterial hemoglobin is 95% saturated and carries 19.8 vol% oxygen. The venous hemoglobin is 75% saturated and carries 15.3 vol% oxygen. Using formula 1, the total amount of midcapillary unoxygenated hemoglobin is 3.3 vol%. Cyanosis *is not* present.

$$\frac{(Co_2 - Cao_2) + (Co_2 - Cvo_2)}{2}$$

Co_2 is hemoglobin fully saturated with oxygen (i.e., Hb in gm/dl × 1.39 cc/100 cc. Hemoglobin, when fully saturated, carries 1.39 cc O_2/100 cc of blood). Cao_2, arterial oxygen content, is Hgb gm/dl × 1.39 × percent actual O_2 saturation in patient's arterial blood. Cvo_2, venous oxygen content, is Hgb gm/dl × 1.39 × patient's actual percent oxygen saturation in venous blood.

CLINICAL ANALYSIS

Five relatively common conditions may be encountered in clinical practice; three of these can produce cyanosis depending on the patient's hemoglobin concentration, the level of Cao_2 and Cvo_2, and cardiac output.

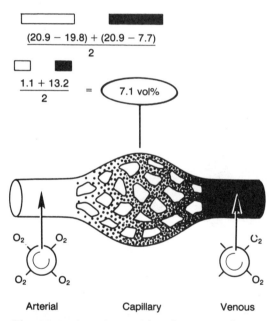

$$\frac{(20.9 - 19.8) + (20.9 - 7.7)}{2}$$

$$\frac{1.1 + 13.2}{2} \quad = \quad \boxed{7.1 \text{ vol\%}}$$

| Arterial | Capillary | Venous |

Fig. 20-2. A patient with a low Cvo_2 due to myocardial dysfunction. The hemoglobin and Cao_2 concentrations are normal, and Cvo_2 is low. The arterial hemoglobin is 95% saturated and carries 19.8 vol% oxygen. The venous hemoglobin is only 35% saturated because of decreased tissue perfusion or increased oxygen extraction. Using formula 1, the amount of unoxygenated hemoglobin at the midcapillary level is 7.1 vol%. Cyanosis is present.

1. Normal patients (Fig. 20–1). The hemoglobin concentration, CaO_2 and CvO_2, and cardiac output are normal at rest and with exercise. Cyanosis does not occur because there is only 3.3 vol% unoxygenated hemoglobin.

2. Patients with a low CvO_2 due to myocardial dysfunction (Fig. 20–2). Cyanosis is present because the total amount of reduced hemoglobin exceeds 5 gm/dl and unoxygenated hemoglobin exceeds 6.95 vol%. This type of cyanosis is classified as *peripheral* and is usually caused by decreased cardiac output or a marked increase in tissue oxygen demands leading to a low CvO_2.

3. Patients with a low CaO_2 due to respiratory disease (Fig. 20–3). *Central* cyanosis is present due to arterial oxygen desaturation. Because the CaO_2 is low, the CvO_2 will necessarily be low even with a normal

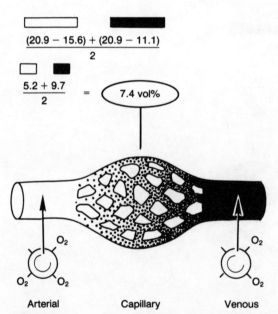

$$\frac{(20.9 - 15.6) + (20.9 - 11.1)}{2}$$

$$\frac{5.2 + 9.7}{2} = \boxed{7.4 \text{ vol\%}}$$

O₂

Arterial   Capillary   Venous

Fig. 20–3. A patient with a low CaO_2 due to respiratory disease. The hemoglobin concentration and cardiac output are normal; CaO_2 and CvO_2 are low. The arterial hemoglobin is only 75% saturated and carries 15.6 vol% of oxygen. Because the arterial oxygen content is low, the venous oxygen content is necessarily low (e.g., 50% saturation). The venous hemoglobin carries 11.1 vol% of oxygen. Using formula 1, the amount of unoxygenated hemoglobin at the midcapillary level is 7.4 vol%. Cyanosis *is* present.

cardiac output. This type of cyanosis is commonly found in patients with respiratory disease when their PaO_2 is less than 40 torr.

4. Patients with polycythemia and low CaO_2 and CvO_2 due to respiratory disease (Fig. 20–4). Cyanosis occurs because more reduced hemoglobin is available at any specific oxygen saturation. The finding of cyanosis in these patients does not imply insufficient oxygen transport to the tissues.

5. Patients with anemia and normal to low CaO_2 and CvO_2 (Figs. 20–5A and 20–5B). Severely anemic patients do not demonstrate cyanosis even when their PvO_2 is very low, as occurs with decreased cardiac output or increased peripheral tissue oxygen demands (Fig. 20–5A). The anemic patient is not cyanotic even with severe arterial oxygen desaturation (Fig. 20–5B).

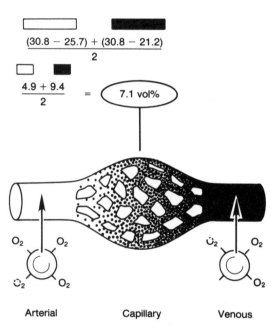

$$\frac{(30.8 - 25.7) + (30.8 - 21.2)}{2}$$

$$\frac{4.9 + 9.4}{2} = \boxed{7.1 \text{ vol\%}}$$

Arterial   Capillary   Venous

Fig. 20–4. A patient with polycythemia and a low CaO_2 and CvO_2 due to respiratory disease. In this example, the hemoglobin concentration is elevated at 22 g/dl. The arterial hemoglobin oxygen saturation is slightly low at 85%. The hemoglobin carries 25.7 vol% of oxygen. The venous hemoglobin is 70% saturated and carries 21.2 vol% of oxygen. Using formula 1, the total unoxygenated hemoglobin at the midcapillary level is 7.1 vol%. Cyanosis *is* present.

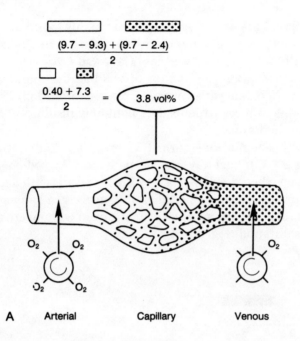

$$\frac{(9.7 - 9.3) + (9.7 - 2.4)}{2}$$

$$\frac{0.40 + 7.3}{2} = \boxed{3.8 \text{ vol\%}}$$

A   Arterial   Capillary   Venous

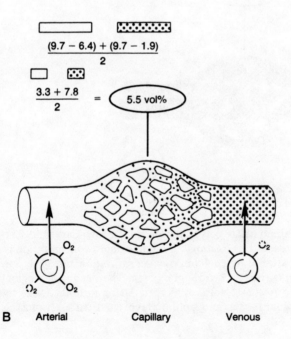

$$\frac{(9.7 - 6.4) + (9.7 - 1.9)}{2}$$

$$\frac{3.3 + 7.8}{2} = \boxed{5.5 \text{ vol\%}}$$

B   Arterial   Capillary   Venous

OTHER FACTORS MODIFYING CYANOSIS

A low $PaCo_2$ (i.e., about 20 torr to 25 torr) causes vasoconstriction that prolongs red blood cell transit time through the peripheral vascular bed. This transit time allows more oxygen to be removed from the hemoglobin per unit time, which lowers the Cvo_2 and accentuates any tendency toward cyanosis. Conversely, hypercapnea causes peripheral vasodilatation with increased cardiac output and shortened transit time and protects against the development of cyanosis.[6]

Detection of cyanosis by the observer also depends on the lighting in the room. Natural lighting with white walls is the best; least desirable is fluorescent lighting with walls of different colors.

NONPULMONARY CAUSES OF CYANOSIS

A variety of abnormal hemoglobins such as methemoglobinemia and sulfhemoglobinemia can cause a cyanotic appearance. Methemoglobinemia, either from hereditary or chemically acquired conditions, decreases the hemoglobin molecule's affinity for binding oxygen and carbon dioxide. The brown-colored pigment of methemoglobin then gives a cyanotic appearance to the skin not corrected by supplemental oxygen administration. Similar to methemoglobinemia, the brown pigment produced by sulfhemoglobin imparts a cyanotic color to the skin.[1,2]

CYANOSIS IN SPECIFIC PULMONARY DISEASES

Although hypoxemia is common in many pulmonary diseases, cyanosis is unusual. The presence of central and peripheral cyanosis in specific pulmonary diseases is listed in the following table. A positive (+) sign indicates cyanosis is relatively common; a negative (−) sign indicates that cyanosis either does not occur or is exceedingly uncommon.

Fig. 20–5. A patient with anemia and a normal Cao_2 and low Cvo_2. A, the hemoglobin is 7.5 g/dl with a normal arterial saturation of 95% and carries 9.3 vol% oxygen. The venous hemoglobin is 25% saturated due to poor tissue perfusion. The oxygen carrying capacity is 2.4 vol%. Using formula 1, there is 3.8 vol% unoxygenated hemoglobin at the midcapillary level. Cyanosis *is not* present. *B*, a patient with anemia and low Cao_2 and Cvo_2. The hemoglobin is 7.5 g/dl. The arterial hemoglobin is 65% saturated and carries 6.4 vol% oxygen. The venous hemoglobin is 20% saturated and carries 1.9 vol% oxygen. Using formula 1, the total amount of unoxygenated hemoglobin at the midcapillary level is 5.5 vol%. Cyanosis *is not* present.

| Disease | Cyanosis | | Comments |
	Central	Peripheral	
Obstructive lung disease			
Common			
2. Chronic bronchitis	+	−	A small percentage of patients, called *blue bloaters*, have arterial desaturations with Pa_{O_2} less than 55 torr and oxygen saturations less than 85%. In addition, if and when cor pulmonale supervenes, a decrease in cardiac output may lead to peripheral oxygen desaturation. The compensatory polycythemia and pulmonary hypertension that can open a patent foramen ovale may rarely contribute to the cyanosis.
3. Asthma	+	−	Central cyanosis appearing during an acute exacerbation is a grave prognostic sign, usually indicating the necessity for immediate intubation and mechanical ventilation.
Uncommon			
4. Bronchiectasis	+	−	Similar to mechanisms in chronic bronchitis.
5. Cystic fibrosis	+	−	Similar to bronchiectasis.
6. Upper airway obstruction	+	−	Profound central cyanosis occurs with sudden and complete upper airway obstruction.
Restrictive lung disease			
Common			
7. Interstitial fibrosis	+	−	Arterial hypoxemia, decreased cardiac output secondary to cor pulmonale, polycythemia, and a patent foramen ovale secondary to pulmonary hypertension may combine to produce cyanosis in advanced disease.
9. Pulmonary edema	+	+	Central and peripheral cyanosis are common in patients with cardiogenic pulmonary edema. This is due to

Disease	Cyanosis		Comments
	Central	Peripheral	
			some combination of arterial desaturation secondary to ventilation perfusion mismatching and decreased cardiac output due to myocardial damage. Hypocapnea with secondary peripheral vasoconstriction can accentuate the cyanosis.
10. Thoracic cage deformities and abnormalities	+	−	Cyanosis occurs with superimposed pneumonias or the onset of chronic respiratory failure.
12. Inhalational or occupational pulmonary diseases	+	−	Cyanosis is common in patients with the acute onset of an alveolar filling process following the inhalation of toxins such as chlorine or nitrogen dioxide.
Uncommon			
14. Goodpasture's syndrome	+	−	Cyanosis depends on the extent of alveolar involvement.
15. Idiopathic hemosiderosis	+	−	Similar to Goodpasture's syndrome.
Pulmonary vascular disease			
Common			
17. Acute pulmonary embolism	+	−	Cyanosis is common in acute massive pulmonary embolism with associated hypotension. It is uncommon with small to moderate size pulmonary emboli.
Uncommon			
18. Sickle cell disease	+	−	Cor pulmonale and ventilation perfusion abnormalities cause cyanosis in a small percentage of patients.
19. Recurrent pulmonary thromboembolism	+	−	Similar to the findings in sickle cell disease.
20. Primary pulmonary hypertension	+	−	Cyanosis is uncommon until the terminal stages of this disease.

	Cyanosis		
Disease	Central	Peripheral	Comments
21. Pulmonary veno-occlusive disease	+	−	Pulmonary edema causes ventilation perfusion mismatching and arterial hypoxemia.

Tumors of the lung, pleura, and mediastinum

Common

22. Carcinoma of the lung	+	−	Cyanosis is uncommon unless postobstruction lobar atelectasis or pneumonia is present.

Infectious diseases of the lung

Common

26. Bacterial, mycoplasmal, and rickettsial pneumonias	+	−	Cyanosis is associated with extensive bilateral disease. Peripheral cyanosis may be due to decreased cardiac output in patients with septic shock.
28. Lung abscesses	+	−	The sudden onset of cyanosis should alert the physician to the possibility of spillage of purulent material into the uninvolved lung.

Uncommon

33. Aspiration lung disease	+	−	Acute upper airway obstruction secondary to foreign body aspiration or bilateral aspiration of fluid can cause cyanosis.
37. Sleep apnea and central hypoventilation syndromes	+	−	Nocturnal cyanosis is common and is due to a combination of arterial hypoxemia and polycythemia.

REFERENCES

1. Fleming PR: Cyanosis. In Hart D (ed): French's Index of Differential Diagnosis, 11th ed, pp 194–199. Chicago, John Wright and Sons, 1979
2. Lukas DS: Cyanosis. In McBryde CM, Blacklow RS (eds): Signs and Symptoms, 5th ed, pp 358–368. Philadelphia, JB Lippincott, 1970
3. Lundsgaard C: Studies on cyanosis: Primary causes of cyanosis. J Exp Med 30:259, 1919
4. Comroe JH: Physiology of Respiration. Chicago, Yearbook Medical Publishers, 1965
5. Lundsgaard C, VanSlyke DD: Cyanosis. Medicine 2:1, 1923

21 · TRACHEAL DEVIATION, PERIPHERAL EDEMA, CHEMOSIS, AND CONJUNCTIVAL VENOUS ENGORGEMENT

JAMES A. THOMPSON III

FREDERICK L. GLAUSER

TRACHEAL DEVIATION

Definition
The trachea is either a midline structure or is normally displaced several millimeters to the right of the midline. Any deviation to the left or further deviation to the right is abnormal.

Detection of Tracheal Deviation and Fixation

Whereas examination of the neck is routinely performed, examination of the trachea is often neglected, and tracheal abnormalities may provide significant clues to the presence of intrathoracic diseases.

The larynx is palpated to evaluate both lateral and upward movement. Laryngeal examination is best done by placing the thumb and index finger on the cricoid cartilage and applying lateral pressure to produce movement (Fig. 21–1). Fixation of the larynx and limitations of lateral movement are most commonly due to laryngeal carcinoma with extension into surrounding tissues. Tracheal fixation due to inflammatory or neoplastic diseases of the mediastinum may freeze the larynx and limit upward movement. In addition, emphysema with a low flat diaphragm may produce downward fixation.[1]

The trachea should be examined with the thumb and index fingers and identified by the presence of the cartilagenous rings. The 4 cm to 5 cm

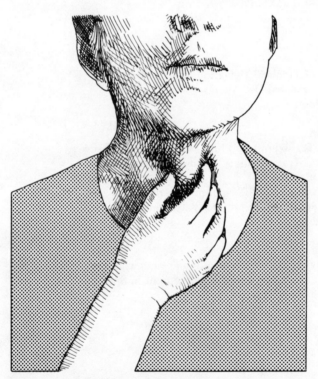

Fig. 21–1. Laryngeal examination. Place the thumb and index finger on the cricoid cartilage and apply lateral pressure to produce movement. Fixation of the larynx can be determined in this fashion.

of trachea between the cricoid cartilage and the suprasternal notch is easily palpated in normal subjects, but may be difficult to palpate in obese patients. Thyroid enlargement may cover or displace the trachea. The best method involves palpation with the tip of the index finger inserted between the sternocleidomastoid muscles to evaluate symmetry and to compare the tracheal position with the midline of the suprasternal notch (Fig. 21–2). Small degrees of tracheal deviation are difficult to detect by physical examination alone.

Causes of Tracheal Deviation

Tracheal deviation may be caused by a cervical mass, goiter, or enlarged lymph nodes located high in the neck. A retrosternal goiter that is eccentrically located below the suprasternal notch may push the trachea to one side. The trachea and mediastinum deviate to the opposite side with massive pleural effusions or a tension pneumothorax. Displacement of the trachea to the ipsilateral side occurs with atelectasis. Bronchial carcinoma causes tracheal displacement from atelectasis secondary to bronchial obstruction.

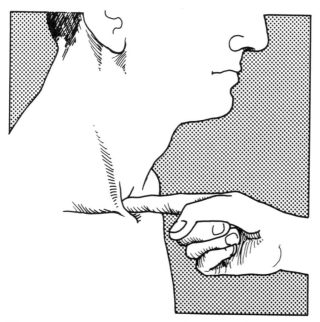

Fig. 21–2. Determination of tracheal deviation. With the tip of the index finger, palpate between the sternocleidomastoid muscles. Evaluate symmetry by comparing the tracheal position to an imaginary line drawn vertically through the suprasternal notch.

PERIPHERAL EDEMA

Definition

Peripheral edema is the accumulation of excess amounts of extracellular or intracellular fluid in peripheral tissues. Edema indicates an alteration in normal physiology and is an important sign of an underlying disease process. Edematous fluid is derived from the circulating blood plasma with a similar composition except for variations in total protein content.

Mechanisms

Normal transcapillary fluid and protein exchange. Fluids and proteins are in dynamic equilibrium between the interstitial, intravascular, and intracellular compartments. Notwithstanding this flux, these compartments remain constant in volume and composition due to multiple interrelated mechanisms. As plasma enters the proximal (arteriolar) end of the capillaries, some fluid exudes into the interstitium because intravascular hydrostatic pressure exceeds colloid osmotic pressure. In the distal (venular) capillary, fluid reenters the intravascular compartment because the interstitial tissue tension and capillary osmotic pressure are higher than capillary hydrostatic pressures.

Small quantities of protein accompany the fluid, which exudes into the interstitium at the arterial end of the capillaries, but when the fluid is resorbed at the venous end, some protein is left behind. Protein progressively accumulates in the interstitial space, in turn increasing the tissue colloid osmotic pressure. This phenomenon decreases resorption of fluid at the terminal end of the capillaries, thereby promoting increased tissue fluid volume and less negative interstitial fluid pressure. These negative pressures allow the lymphatics to pump this proteinacious interstitial fluid into the venous system, thus returning the excess proteins to the circulatory system.[2]

Factors that lead to the formation of edema compromise one or more of the normal functions governing the exchange of fluid between the compartments. Simultaneous or sequential alterations in several of these factors are possible in patients with pulmonary disease.

Abnormal transcapillary fluid and protein exchange. Increased Capillary Permeability. Increased peripheral capillary permeability is usually associated with pulmonary vasculitides, acute infections, connective tissue diseases, and some forms of the acute respiratory distress syndrome.

Increased Capillary Hydrostatic Pressure. Peripheral edema due to increased capillary hydrostatic pressure is found in disease states that increase venous pressure, thereby decreasing fluid resorption in the distal capillary.

The increased pressure is usually secondary to either local factors such as venous obstruction from tumor or clot or to an increase in central venous pressure. The causes of the central venous pressure elevation are numerous, but it generally results from right atrial and ventricular pressure increases secondary to pulmonary hypertension.

Decreased Intravascular Colloid Osmotic Pressure. A decrease in colloid osmotic pressure is usually secondary to a loss of protein from the intravascular compartment; therefore, any chronic or severe debilitating state such as a malignancy or a chronic inflammatory disease will cause a low oncotic pressure. This increases the amount of fluid exuding from the capillaries into the interstitial space.

Increased Interstitial Colloid Osmotic Pressure and Lymphatic Obstruction. An increase in interstitial colloid osmotic pressure due to an increase in capillary permeability or a decrease in lymphatic flow results in the accumulation of interstitial protein and fluid. A decrease in mechanical interstitial pressures resulting in edema is seen in elderly people with low elastic tissue forces and in chronically protein-malnourished patients. In addition, lymphatic obstruction results in a high protein fluid in the interstitium with resultant edema. Lymphatic insufficiency may be caused by primary tumors, metastatic compression, or occasionally by fibrosis secondary to chronic infection.

Clinical Evaluation of Peripheral Edema

Both the distribution and the depth or thickness of any edema found should be recorded. Edema may be either localized or generalized. Body weight may increase by 10% or more before generalized edema is found on physical examination.

Dependent edema first appears in the ankles and feet in ambulatory patients. Patients confined to bed may exhibit edema only on the posterior surface of the sacrum (sacral edema) or backs of the legs. The subcutaneous tissues and the skin become fibrotic (brawny edema), and pitting can no longer be found when edema has been present for a long period of time.

The localization of the edema may be a clue to a specific diagnosis. Unilateral edema of a lower extremity in a patient with acute shortness of breath may be due to venous thrombosis causing pulmonary embolism. Pancoast's tumor of the lung may lead to unilateral upper extremity edema. Bilateral upper extremity and facial swelling with suffusion and neck vein distention is found in the superior vena cava syndrome. A large majority of these cases are due to carcinoma of the lung.

Edema is unusual during the early stages of chronic bronchitis; it is common when cor pulmonale develops with resultant right ventricular failure. Patients with sleep apnea syndrome or primary hypoventilation occasionally develop pedal edema secondary to cor pulmonale and right heart failure.[3] Patients with scoliosis experience edema formation when chronic respiratory failure and cor pulmonale supervene. Peripheral edema is uncommon in most patients with acute pulmonary diseases unless there is a concomitant increase in vascular permeability as in overwhelming sepsis. In general, edema is not a prominent finding in acute bacterial, viral, or fungal pneumonias.

It is uncommon for an asthmatic patient to have edema unless underlying severe chronic obstructive lung disease (chronic bronchitis) is present. Congestive heart failure, pulmonary embolism, or bronchial obstruction should be suspected in patients who wheeze and have peripheral edema. In a young woman with severe dyspnea on exertion and peripheral edema, the diagnosis of chronic recurrent pulmonary emboli or primary pulmonary hypertension should be considered.[4]

Occupational lung diseases, asbestosis, and silicosis, when advanced, may be associated with edema secondary to cor pulmonale. Patients with advanced interstitial lung disease, including sarcoidosis, may have edema when pulmonary hypertension supervenes. A patient with massive edema will occasionally have a past history of tuberculosis; diagnosis of constrictive pericarditis should be considered.

BILATERAL CHEMOSIS AND CONJUNCTIVAL VENOUS ENGORGEMENT

Definition
Chemosis is defined as ocular conjunctival edema that forms a swelling around the cornea. Venous engorgement is distention of conjunctival vessels, which imparts a reddish color to the cornea.

Mechanisms
Papilledema and retinopathy are well-known complications of certain forms of pulmonary disease.[5] Patients with superimposed acute and chronic respiratory failure have been reported to present with bilateral chemosis and conjunctival venous engorgement associated with jugular venous distention, peripheral edema, hypoxemia, and hypercapnea. Most of these patients had chronic obstructive pulmonary disease, usually chronic bronchitis, with right

and left ventricular failure; a minority had idiopathic pulmonary fibrosis with cor pulmonale.[6]

The cause of the chemosis and conjunctival venous engorgement is unclear, but they may be due to a variety of factors including the following:

Increased venous pressure. The conjunctival venous system empties into the cavenous sinus at the posterior orbit. This vessel connects with the saggittal sinus and drains into the internal jugular vein, which eventually connects to the superior vena cava by way of the common jugular. A rich lymphatic network also drains the con-junctivae. These channels empty into the venous system after pass-ing through the submaxillary lymphatic chain. The conjunctival vasculature can therefore be exposed to the increased pressures gen-erated in the right side of the heart such as occur in patients with cor pulmonale and right ventricular failure.

The effects of hypoxemia on retinal and conjunctival vasculature. Hypoxemia can dilate both retinal and conjunctival vessels. Patients with cystic fibrosis and hypoxemia may have retinal changes in-cluding venous engorgement, macular edema, retinal hemorrhages, and papilledema.

Hypercapnea. Hypercapnea has also been implicated in retinal vas-cular dilatation.

Most patients with bilateral chemosis and conjunctival venous en-gorgement have right ventricular failure with elevated jugular venous pressure in addition to hypoxemia and hypercapnea. A combination of events is prob-ably necessary for patients to manifest this ocular sign.

TRACHEAL DEVIATION, PERIPHERAL EDEMA, CHEMOSIS, AND CONJUNCTIVAL VENOUS ENGORGEMENT IN SPECIFIC PULMONARY DISEASES

The following table lists the presence of tracheal deviation, peripheral edema, chemosis, and conjunctival venous engorgement in specific pulmonary diseases. A positive (+) sign indicates that the specific physical sign may be present; a negative (−) sign indicates that the sign either does not occur or is quite uncommon in a specific pulmonary disease.

Disease	Tracheal deviation	Peripheral edema	Chemosis and conjunctival venous engorgement	Comments
Obstructive lung disease				
Common				
2. Chronic bronchitis	−	+	+	Peripheral edema is found in patients with advanced disease and cor pulmonale. Biventricular failure is common.
Uncommon				
4. Bronchiectasis	−	+	+	Advanced disease is associated with cor pulmonale that leads to peripheral edema.
5. Cystic fibrosis	−	+	+	Similar to bronchiectasis.
6. Upper airway obstruction	+	+	−	Upper airway obstruction from tumors or masses may cause tracheal deviation. Peripheral edema occurs in patients with chronic hypercapnea, hypoxemia, and cor pulmonale.
Restrictive lung disease				
Common				
9. Pulmonary edema	−	+	−	Patients with left ventricular failure may also have right ventricular failure with peripheral edema.
10. Thoracic cage deformities and abnormalities	+	−	−	Deformity of the thoracic cage can secondarily lead to tracheal deviation.

Disease	Tracheal deviation	Peripheral edema	Chemosis and conjunctival venous engorgement	Comments
Pulmonary vascular disease				
Common				
11. Acute pulmonary embolism	–	+	–	Patients with large emboli may have acute cor pulmonale and peripheral edema. Peripheral venous thrombosis can also cause peripheral edema.
19. Recurrent pulmonary thromboembolism	–	+	–	Peripheral edema is one of the most common physical findings in this disease.
20. Primary pulmonary hypertension	–	+	–	Similar to recurrent pulmonary thromboembolism.
21. Pulmonary veno-occlusive disease	–	+	–	Similar to recurrent pulmonary thromboembolism.
Tumors of the lung, pleura, and mediastinum				
Common				
22. Carcinoma of the lung	+	–	–	Tracheal deviation may be due to the tumor impinging on the trachea or major bronchi. Lobar or whole lung atelectasis can cause tracheal deviation.
Uncommon				
24. Malignant mesothelioma	+	–	–	The trachea may be deviated away from the side of the pleural effusion or thickening.

Disease	Tracheal deviation	Peripheral edema	Chemosis and conjunctival venous engorgement	Comments
25. Bronchial adenomas	+	–	–	Tracheal deviation will occur toward the side of the lesion with lobar or whole lung atelectasis.
Miscellaneous				
36. Sleep apnea and central hypoventilation syndrome	–	+	+	Cor pulmonale and right ventricular failure are common in advanced disease.

REFERENCES

1. Stubbing DG, Mathur PN, Roberts RS et al: Some physical signs in patients with chronic airway obstruction. Am Rev Respir Dis 125:549–552, 1982
2. Wallace AG: Clinical manifestations of heart failure. In Beeson PB, McDermott W, Wyngaarden JB (eds): Cecil's Textbook of Medicine, 15th ed, p 1092. Philadelphia, W B Saunders, 1979
3. Guilleninault TC, van der Hoed J, Mitler N: Clinical overview of the sleep apnea syndromes. In Guilleninault C, Dement WC (eds): Sleep Apnea Syndrome, pp 1–12. New York, Allan R. Liss, 1978
4. Wagenvoort CA, Wagenvoort N: Primary pulmonary hypertension. A pathological study of the lung vessels in 156 clinically diagnosed cases. Circulation 42:1163, 1970
5. Simpson T: Papilledema and emphysema. Br Med J 2:639, 1948
6. Glauser FL: Bilateral chemosis and conjunctival venous engorgement in cardiopulmonary failure. Chest 66:389, 1974

part III
SPECIFIC DISEASES

22 · CLINICAL AND LABORATORY FINDINGS IN SPECIFIC PULMONARY DISEASES

FREDERICK L. GLAUSER

Emphysema
Chronic Bronchitis
Asthma
Bronchiectasis
Cystic Fibrosis
Upper Airway Obstruction
Interstitial Fibrosis
Sarcoidosis
Pulmonary Edema
Thoracic Cage Deformities and Abnormalities
Neuromuscular Disorders
Inhalational or Occupational Pulmonary Diseases
Hypersensitivity Pneumonitis
Goodpasture's Syndrome
Idiopathic Pulmonary Hemosiderosis
Eosinophilic Granuloma
Acute Pulmonary Embolism
Sickle Cell Disease
Recurrent Pulmonary Thromboembolism
Primary Pulmonary Hypertension
Pulmonary Veno-occlusive Disease
Carcinoma of the Lung
Metastatic Carcinoma of the Lung
Malignant Mesothelioma
Bronchial Adenomas
Bacterial, Mycoplasmal, and Rickettsial Pneumonias
Viral Pneumonias
Lung Abscesses
Tuberculosis
Atypical Tuberculosis
Actinomyces and *Nocardia*
Mycoses

Aspiration Lung Disease
Pulmonary Alveolar Proteinosis
Wegener's Granulomatosis, Its Variants, and Other
        Vasculitides
Sleep Apnea and Central Hypoventilation Syndromes

In order for the reader to correctly identify the diseases discussed in the text, this chapter presents definitions, laboratory findings, chest radiograph appearance, electrocardiographic changes, arterial blood gases, and pulmonary function tests for each specific pulmonary disease. The numbers beside each disease are the same as those used throughout the text. The descriptions presented here are of the most common findings in moderately advanced diseases. Unusual, atypical, or advanced aspects of these diseases *are not* covered. Standard pulmonary textbooks should be consulted for more detailed information.

EMPHYSEMA (1)

Emphysema is characterized by the silent, progressive destruction of pulmonary alveoli and capillaries with eventual coalescence of multiple alveoli. This disease is related to cigarette smoking, with symptoms beginning at the age of 45 to 55 years.

> *Laboratory*—No characteristic findings.
> *Chest Radiograph*—Hyperlucent and overexpanded lung fields; small narrow "vertical" heart; increased anteroposterior diameter of the chest; low flat diaphragm. Apical bullae are common; basilar bullae or hyperlucency suggest the diagnosis of α-1 antitrypsin deficiency.
> *Electrocardiogram*—Low voltage; right axis deviation.
> *Arterial Blood Gases*—PaO_2, greater than 55 torr; $PaCO_2$, 30 torr to 40 torr; pH, normal.
> *Pulmonary Function Tests*—Lung volumes are normal or increased; flow rates are decreased; diffusing capacity for CO (DLCO) is low. No response to bronchodilators.[1,2]

CHRONIC BRONCHITIS (2)

Chronic bronchitis is pathologically characterized by mucus gland hypertrophy and increased sputum production. Patients complain of a chronic productive cough for 2 to 3 months out of the year for 2 years in a row. Cough and sputum production are related to cigarette smoking. Symptoms begin at 45 to 55 years of age.

Laboratory—Sputum eosinophils and blood eosinophila occur. Polycythemia is present in patients with chronic hypoxemia.

Chest Radiograph—Increased bibasilar, peribronchial markings with a normal-sized heart.

Electrocardiogram—Normal or evidence of right ventricular strain.

Arterial Blood Gases—Similar to levels in patients with emphysema. Approximately 10% of patients experience hypoxemia (PaO$_2$ less than 55 torr), hypercapnea (PaCO$_2$ greater than 45 torr), and a compensated respiratory acidosis (pH of 7.32 to 7.38).

Pulmonary Function Tests—Lung volumes are normal; flow rates decreased; DLCO is slightly low or normal. There may be marked improvement in the flow rates with administration of bronchodilators.[2]

ASTHMA (3)

An episodic and reversible disease of large and small airways, asthma is characterized by bronchospasm, mucosal edema, and increased sputum production. Asthma can be arbitrarily subclassified into two types: extrinsic (atopic), in which a history of allergy exists, and intrinsic, in which no allergic component is present. Most of the patients in the extrinsic category are younger than 15 years, whereas those in the intrinsic category are older than 25 to 30 years.

Laboratory—Sputum eosinophils and blood eosinophilia are common. Serum IgE levels are elevated in patients with extrinsic asthma.

Chest Radiograph—Normal between attacks; hyperinflation with attacks; 3% of asthmatics experience pneumothoraces.

Electrocardiogram—Normal between attacks; low voltage and P pulmonale may be seen during severe attacks.

Arterial Blood Gases—Mild hypoxemia and hypocapnea are common between attacks and worsen with moderate attacks. Normocapnea and hypercapnea occur with severe attacks.

Pulmonary Function Tests—Lung volumes are normal or increased; flow rates are decreased; DLCO is normal or increased. Administration of bronchodilators leads to significant improvement in flow rates or vital capacity.[3]

BRONCHIECTASIS (4)

Bronchiectasis is characterized by pathologic dilation of the bronchi with destruction of bronchial walls. A multitude of etiologies and diseases are associated with bronchiectasis, including repeated or prolonged episodes of necrotizing pneumonitis; bronchial obstruction due to neoplasm, lymph nodes, or a foreign body; genetic or developmental causes; cystic fibrosis; dysfunctional or immotile cilia syndrome; agammaglobulinemia; traction bronchiectasis secondary to localized pulmonary fibrosis; and bronchopulmonary aspergillosis.

Laboratory—Anemia of chronic disease is common. Staphylococcus, streptococcus, and pseudomonas are commonly identified on sputum smears and cultures.

Chest Radiograph—Usually normal; air fluid levels and fibronodular infiltrates interspersed with cystic areas may be found in advanced, diffuse disease; heart size is usually normal.

Electrocardiogram—Usually normal but may reveal evidence of cor pulmonale.

Arterial Blood Gases—Mild hypoxemia and hypocapnea are common.

Pulmonary Function Tests—Lung volumes normal or slightly decreased; flow rates are decreased; DLCO is normal or slightly low. Airway obstruction may respond to administration of bronchodilators.[4]

CYSTIC FIBROSIS (5)

Cystic fibrosis is a hereditary disorder characterized by dysfunction of the exocrine glands throughout the body and presents as a triad of chronic pulmonary disease, pancreatic insufficiency, and abnormally high sweat chloride levels. The lung disease is a form of bronchiectasis with predilection for the upper lobes. Patients are prone to chronic, recurrent pulmonary infections, and respiratory insufficiency supervenes at a relatively young age.

Laboratory—The anemia of chronic disease is common. Sweat chloride levels higher than 80 mEq/liter to 100 mEq/liter are diagnostic.

Chest Radiograph—Increased peribronchial markings and interstitial infiltrates with a predilection for the upper lobes are characteristic; heart size is normal.

Electrocardiogram—Usually normal but may reveal evidence of cor pulmonale.

Arterial Blood Gases—Hypoxemia and mild hypocapnea are common.

Pulmonary Function Tests—Similar to those found with bronchiectasis.[5]

UPPER AIRWAY OBSTRUCTION (6)

Upper airway obstruction is a physiologic and pathologic abnormality caused by a variety of diseases. Some causes of upper airway obstruction are as follows:

1. Oropharyngeal obstruction
    Enlarged tonsils and adenoids; micronathia
    Enlarged tongue (e.g., acromegaly, hypothyroidism)
    Epiglottic edema secondary to trauma, allergies, or C1 esterase deficiency
2. Intrathoracic and extrathoracic tracheal obstruction
    Enlarged thyroid
    Intrinsic or extrinsic compressing tumors
    Tracheolaryngeal edema, tumors, polyps
    Foreign body
    Trauma
3. Large bronchi
    Airway tumors
    External compression from tumors, fibrosis, lymph nodes
    Trauma

Inspiratory wheezing or stridor is common in patients with symptomatic extrathoracic tracheal airway obstruction. Conversely, patients with intrathoracic tracheal or major bronchial obstruction experience expiratory wheezing. The stridor and wheeze may not be obvious until maximum inspiratory and expiratory maneuvers are performed. Chronic upper airway obstruction may cause chronic hypercapnea and hypoxemia eventuating in pulmonary hypertension and cor pulmonale. Many patients with chronic upper airway obstruction are misdiagnosed as suffering from COPD.

Laboratory—Polycythemia may be present in patients with chronic hypoxemia.

Chest Radiograph—Usually normal; there may be evidence of tracheal compression.

Electrocardiogram—Usually normal.

Arterial Blood Gases—With mild disease, arterial blood gases are normal; with severe, advanced obstruction hypercapnea is common.

Pulmonary Function Tests—Lung volumes are normal; flow rates are minimally decreased; DLCO is normal. Flow volume loops reveal a plateau of flow during inspiration or expiration, depending on the site of obstruction (Figs. 15–3 and 15–4).

Miscellaneous—Tracheal tomography and bronchoscopy may be helpful in establishing the diagnosis.[6]

INTERSTITIAL FIBROSIS (7)

A multitude of entities can eventuate in interstitial fibrosis:

1. Idiopathic or primary
   UIP—usual interstitial pneumonitis, cryptogenic fibrosing alveolitis, chronic interstitial fibrosis
   Desquamative interstitial pneumonitis
   Lymphocytic interstitial pneumonitis
2. Secondary
   Part of a multisystem disease (e.g., systemic lupus erythematosis, rheumatoid arthritis, etc.)
   Drug induced—bleomycin, nitrofuradantoin, and so on
   Secondary to dust inhalation
   Secondary to noxious fumes
   Adult respiratory distress syndrome, advanced
   Oxygen toxicity
   Paraquat poisoning
   Radiation fibrosis
   Sarcoidosis

Classically, the patient has a restrictive type of lung disease and lung biopsy reveals both interstitial and interalveolar fibrosis. Lung compliance is decreased but the airways are usually not affected.

Laboratory—Anemia is common; serum immune complexes, lupus erythematosus preparations, rheumatoid factors, and antinuclear antibodies may be positive.

Chest Radiograph—Lung fields appear small; diaphragms are elevated; increased interstitial markings either localized to the bases or diffusely affecting the lungs; in 6% of patients, the chest radiograph is normal.

Electrocardiogram—Normal.

Arterial Blood Gases—Mild hypoxemia (PaO_2 higher than 55 torr) and hypocapnea ($PaCO_2$ about 30 torr to 35 torr) are common.

Pulmonary Function Tests—Lung volumes are decreased; flow rates are normal; DLCO is low.

Miscellaneous—Transbronchial or open lung biopsy may be necessary to establish the diagnosis. During active disease bronchoalveolar lavage may reveal an increased number of neutrophils.[7]

SARCOIDOSIS (8)

Sarcoidosis is a multisystemic granulomatous disorder of unknown etiology presenting most frequently in young adults with bilateral hilar lymphadenopathy, pulmonary infiltrates, and skin and eye lesions. Abnormal function of both lung lymphocytes and macrophages appear to play a key role in the pathogenesis, although the etiology of the lung disease remains obscure.

Laboratory—Anemia of chronic disease may be present. Hypergammaglobulin is common. Hypercalcemia occurs in 10% of patients although hypercalciuria is common.

Chest Radiograph—The four classic patterns are bilateral hilar adenopathy with clear lung fields, bilateral hilar adenopathy with interstitial infiltrates, interstitial infiltrates without adenopathy, and progressive massive fibrosis with cystic changes. Pleural effusions are uncommon.

Electrocardiogram—Usually normal. Conduction defects and arrythmias are found in myocardial sarcoidosis.

Arterial Blood Gases—Mild resting hypoxemia worsening with exercise is common.

Pulmonary Function Tests—Lung volumes are normal or decreased; flow rates are normal; DLCO is decreased.

Miscellaneous—Gallium lung scans may be positive; serum angiotensin-converting enzyme (ACE) levels are commonly elevated.[8]

PULMONARY EDEMA (9)

Pulmonary edema is defined as an increase in lung water secondary to increased pulmonary capillary hydrostatic pressure, as in cardiogenic pulmonary edema, and increased alveolar capillary membrane permeability, as in the adult respiratory distress syndrome. Cardiogenic pulmonary edema is characterized by low protein concentrations in the pulmonary edema fluid in contrast to increased permeability pulmonary edema, in which the protein concentrations are elevated.

Laboratory—No characteristic findings.

Chest Radiograph—Bilateral interstitial and alveolar infiltrates are found in both forms of pulmonary edema; the heart may be enlarged in patients with cardiogenic pulmonary edema; Kerley's lines are common in patients with chronic cardiogenic pulmonary edema.

Electrocardiogram—Varies depending on the disease process; in patients with cardiogenic pulmonary edema, there may be evidence of an old or recent myocardial infarction; in these patients arrythmias are common.

Arterial Blood Gases—Hypoxemia and hypocapnea are common in both forms of pulmonary edema.

Pulmonary Function Tests—Lung volumes are normal or decreased; flow rates are usually normal; DLCO is normal or low.[9]

THORACIC CAGE DEFORMITIES AND ABNORMALITIES (10)

These diseases include patients with scoliosis, kyphoscoliosis, fibrothorax, thoracoplasty, and ankylosing spondylitis. Physiologically, these disorders have the following in common: ventilation perfusion mismatching secondary to lung compression from the deformed thoracic cage, an ineffective cough due to expiratory muscle disadvantage, and increased work of breathing secondary to the mechanical abnormalities of the chest wall.

Laboratory—Anemia is common.

Chest Radiograph—The film is distinctive depending on the specific disease process.

Electrocardiogram—Usually normal.

Arterial Blood Gases—Hypoxemia is common.

Pulmonary Function Tests—Lung volumes are normal or decreased; flow rates are normal; DLCO is normal or decreased.[10]

NEUROMUSCULAR DISORDERS (11)

Postpoliomyelitis, amytrophic lateral sclerosis, muscular dystrophies, spinal cord injuries, multiple sclerosis, and myasthenia gravis are the most common neuromuscular diseases affecting the lungs. Respiratory failure is common in all of these diseases except for multiple sclerosis.

Laboratory—Anemia of chronic disease is common.

Chest Radiograph—Clear, with elevated diaphragms.

Electrocardiogram—Normal.

Arterial Blood Gases—Hypoxemia with hypocapnea or normocapnea is common. As the diseases progress and muscular weakness worsens, hypercapnea ensues.

Pulmonary Function Tests—Lung volumes are normal or decreased; flow rates are decreased; DLCO is normal or low.[10]

INHALATIONAL OR OCCUPATIONAL PULMONARY DISEASES (12)

These diseases can be classified into those caused by inhalation of inorganic dust such as silica or asbestos (leading to pulmonary fibrosis); organic dust, which causes hypersensitivity pneumonitis (see below); chemicals, fumes, and vapors such as chlorine, nitrogen dioxide, and methane, which can lead to several reactions including acute pulmonary edema, bronchospasm, and acute and chronic bronchitis.

Laboratory—Usually not helpful.

Chest Radiograph—A variety of patterns are seen, including normal patterns, hyperinflation in patients with asthmalike reactions, bilateral interstitial and alveolar infiltrates in patients with acute pulmonary edema, and fibronodular and fibrotic reactions from the inhalation of dusts.

Electrocardiogram—Normal.

Arterial Blood Gases—Varies from normal to mild hypoxemia and hypocapnea.

Pulmonary Function Tests—In patients with inhalation of inorganic dusts and with pulmonary edemalike reactions, lung volumes are decreased, flow rates are normal, DLCO is normal or low. Patients with asthmalike reaction or acute bronchitis have normal or increased lung volumes, decreased flow rates, and a normal DLCO.[11]

HYPERSENSITIVITY PNEUMONITIS (13)

Hypersensitivity pneumonitis is one of the more common types of inhalational or occupational pulmonary diseases. Subtypes are as follows:

1. Farmers' lung
2. Bagassosis
3. Sequoiosis

4. Cheese workers' lung
5. Bird Breeders' lung
6. Pituitary snuff lung
7. Paprika splitters' lung
8. Maple bark strippers' lung
9. Humidifier or air conditioner lung

The inhalation of organic dusts or fungi causes an antigen antibody reaction mainly confined to the lungs. This reaction leads to increased permeability of the alveolar capillary membrane with an influx of plasma and inflammatory cells into the alveolus. The pulmonary pathology reverses with removal of the offending organism; however, in a small percentage of patients, continual exposure to the inhaled antigen may lead to interstitial fibrosis. Inhalation of the offending antigen also causes bronchospasm in a minority of patients.

Laboratory—Leukocytosis and eosinophilia are common; the sedimentation rate is elevated.

Chest Radiograph—During the acute attack, bilateral interstitial and alveolar infiltrates with a normal heart size are common.

Electrocardiogram—Normal.

Arterial Blood Gases—Hypoxemia and hypocapnea are common during attacks.

Pulmonary Function Tests—Lung volumes are normal or decreased; flow rates may be decreased; DLCO is normal or low. The obstructive component may respond to the administration of bronchodilators.

Miscellaneous—Serum precipitins to the specific fungi are positive; serum IgE levels may be elevated.[12]

GOODPASTURE'S SYNDROME (14)

Goodpasture's syndrome is found in patients over 20 years of age who have a combination of hemoptysis, pulmonary infiltrates, and hematuria. Circulating antibodies and complement damage the pulmonary and renal vascular endothelium resulting in glomerulonephritis and pulmonary hemorrhage.

Laboratory—Anemia is common due to renal and pulmonary bleeding. Hemosiderin-laden macrophages in the sputum and hematuria are characteristic. Elevated serum BUN and creatinine are found with renal failure.

Chest Radiograph—Bilateral alveolar infiltrates with a normal heart size are common.

Electrocardiogram—Normal.

Arterial Blood Gases—Varying degrees of hypoxemia and hypocapnea are common.

Pulmonary Function Tests—Lung volumes are normal or decreased; flow rates are normal; DLCO may be inappropriately elevated.

Miscellaneous—Serum antiglomerular basement membrane antibodies are positive. Lung or kidney biopsies reveal positive basement membrane immunofluorescence for complement and IgG antibodies.[13]

IDIOPATHIC PULMONARY HEMOSIDEROSIS (15)

This is a disease of children and young adults under 20 years of age. It is characterized by pulmonary infiltrates and a microcytic hypochromic iron deficiency anemia. Chronic and recurrent extravasation of blood into the pulmonary tissues leads to long-term, low-grade inflammation eventuating in fibrosis.

Laboratory—Microcytic hypochromic anemia is common; sputum reveals hemosiderin laden macrophages.

Chest Radiograph—Bilateral interstitial or alveolar infiltrates are characteristic.

Electrocardiogram—Normal.

Arterial Blood Gases—Hypocapnea and hypoxemia are common.

Pulmonary Function Tests—Lung volumes are normal or low; flow rates are normal; DLCO is normal or elevated.[13]

EOSINOPHILIC GRANULOMA (16)

This is a disease of young adult men and is either confined to the lungs or involves bone, brain, and endocrine organs as well as spleen, liver, and lymph nodes. Interstitial infiltrates comprised of histiocytes, macrophages, and eosinophils that form granulomas affect the lung diffusely.

Laboratory—No characteristic findings.

Chest Radiograph—Diffuse interstitial or fibronodular infiltrates with cystic areas; lung volumes are preserved; spontaneous pneumothorax is common.

Electrocardiogram—Normal.

Arterial Blood Gases—Hypoxemia and hypocapnea are common.
Pulmonary Function Tests—Lung volumes are normal; flow rates are normal; DLCO is normal or low.[14]

ACUTE PULMONARY EMBOLISM (17)

Pulmonary embolus denotes the passage of a venous thrombus into the pulmonary artery leading to complete or partial vascular obstruction. Most commonly, thrombi form in the deep veins of the lower extremities. The pelvic veins and the right side of the heart can also be the source of the embolus. Fewer than 10% of pulmonary embolic events result in infarction. The three factors that predispose toward venous thrombosis are venous stasis, damage to the venous endothelial lining, and increased blood coagulability (e.g., hypercoagulability). Certain patients are at increased risk for developing pulmonary embolism.

> *Laboratory*—No characteristic findings.
> *Chest Radiograph*—In over 90% of patients with pulmonary embolus, the chest radiograph is abnormal, showing some combination of elevated diaphragms, platelike atelectasis, hyperlucent lung fields, small pleural effusions, or interstitial infiltrates.
> *Electrocardiogram*—Usually normal. In patients with large pulmonary emboli and systemic hypotension, a right ventricular strain pattern may be present.
> *Arterial Blood Gases*—Hypoxemia and hypocapnea are common.
> *Pulmonary Function Tests*—Lung volumes are normal; flow rates are normal; DLCO is normal or low.
> *Miscellaneous*—Ventilation perfusion scans, venography, ^{131}I-fibrinogen uptake studies and plethysmography may be helpful in establishing a diagnosis. The standard for diagnosis is performance of pulmonary angiography.[15,16]

SICKLE CELL DISEASE (18)

This disease is caused by homozygosity for hemoglobin S and consists of unrelenting hemolytic anemia, recurrent episodes of abdominal and limb pain, and fever with multiorgan involvement. *In situ* pulmonary vascular thrombosis eventuates in pulmonary hypertension and cor pulmonale. Recurrent pneumococcal pneumonias are common.

Laboratory—Anemia is universal. Electrophoretic analysis of blood reveals the characteristic hemoglobin S.

Chest Radiograph—May vary from normal to diffuse bilateral interstitial infiltrates; pneumonias and pulmonary infarctions are characterized by subsegmental or lobar infiltrates; pleural effusions are common.

Electrocardiogram—Normal.

Arterial Blood Gases—Hypoxemia and hypocapnea are common.

Pulmonary Function Tests—Lung volumes are normal or decreased; flow rates are normal; DLCO is low.[17]

RECURRENT PULMONARY THROMBOEMBOLISM (19)

This is a rare but well-recognized cause of chronic pulmonary hypertension. The emboli usually arise from thrombi formed in the iliofemoral system. Over months or years, these emboli gradually obstruct the pulmonary arterial system. Patients usually present with signs of cor pulmonale.

Laboratory—Not helpful.

Chest Radiograph—Lung fields are clear with enlarged right ventricle and atrium.

Electrocardiogram—When cor pulmonale supervenes, evidence of right ventricular hypertrophy and strain are present.

Arterial Blood Gases—Hypoxemia either at rest or with exercise is universal; hypocapnea is common.

Pulmonary Function Tests—Lung volumes are normal; flow rates are normal; DLCO is low.

Miscellaneous—Ventilation perfusion scans and pulmonary angiograms are helpful in establishing the diagnosis.[15,16]

PRIMARY PULMONARY HYPERTENSION (20)

This disease of unknown etiology predominates in middle-aged women. It is relentlessly progressive and refractory to all forms of therapy. Death supervenes approximately 5 years after the onset of symptoms.

Laboratory—Not helpful.

Chest Radiograph—Clear lung fields with evidence of right ventricular enlargement.

Electrocardiogram—Consistent with cor pulmonale.

Arterial Blood Gases—Hypoxemia and hypocapnea are common.

Pulmonary Function Tests—Lung volumes are normal; flow rates are normal; DLCO is low.

Miscellaneous—Ventilation perfusion scans may be normal. Pulmonary angiograms and right heart catheterization may suggest the diagnosis. Open lung biopsy is necessary to identify the characteristic plexiform changes in the pulmonary arteries.[16]

PULMONARY VENO-OCCLUSIVE DISEASE (21)

This rare disease of unknown etiology is characterized by widespread fibrotic narrowing of small and medium-sized pulmonary veins. Patients experience recurrent episodes of pulmonary edema or pulmonary infarction. Death usually occurs within 1 year of the onset of symptoms.

Laboratory—Not helpful.

Chest Radiograph—Bilateral interstitial or alveolar infiltrates consistent with pulmonary edema are common.

Electrocardiogram—Usually normal.

Arterial Blood Gases—Hypoxemia and hypocapnea are common.

Pulmonary Function Tests—Lung volumes are normal or low; flow rates are normal: DLCO is normal or low.[16]

CARCINOMA OF THE LUNG (22)

Carcinoma of the lung can be classified histiologically as epidermoid or squamous cell, small cell, adenocarcinoma, and large cell. Most of these forms of lung carcinoma are caused by or related to cigarette smoking. The incidence of carcinoma of the lung is highest during the sixth decade in men and the seventh decade in women.

Laboratory—Anemia is common. Because many of these tumors secrete hormonally active substances, hyponatremia (inappropriate ADH), hypercalcemia (from bone metastases, parathyroidlike hormone, or prostaglandin secretion), and hypokalemic alkalosis (from increased secretion of ACTH) are common.

Chest Radiograph—Central and peripheral masses with hilar enlargement are common; pleural effusions, elevated diaphragms from phrenic nerve paralysis, and post-obstructive pneumonias are also common.

Electrocardiogram—Usually normal.

Arterial Blood Gases—Hypoxemia and hypocapnea are common, either due to parenchymal involvement by the tumor or the underlying chronic lung disease.

Pulmonary Function Tests—No characteristic pulmonary function findings in carcinoma of the lung. Abnormalities may reflect the presence of underlying chronic lung disease.

Miscellaneous—Sputum cytology, bronchoscopy, mediastinotomy, and thoracotomy in addition to liver, bone, and brain scans, where indicated, may establish the diagnosis.[18]

METASTATIC CARCINOMA
OF THE LUNG (23)

Tumors that frequently metastasize to the lung include malignant melanoma, renal and testicular carcinomas, and breast and contralateral lung tumors. Thirty to forty percent of patients dying of extrathoracic malignant tumors experience pulmonary metastases. These tumors can metastasize to the parenchyma, pleura, or intrabronchial regions.

Laboratory—Findings reflect the source and subtype of the underlying tumor.

Chest Radiograph—Variable findings including solitary or multiple discrete nodules, diffuse or localized infiltrates, hilar or mediastinal lymph node enlargement, and pleural effusions.

Electrocardiogram—Normal.

Arterial Blood Gases—Hypoxemia depends on the extent of pulmonary involvement.

Pulmonary Function Tests—Nonspecific and nondiagnostic.

Miscellaneous—Sputum cytology, bronchoscopy, and thoracentesis confirm the diagnosis in 20% to 40% of cases.[19]

MALIGNANT MESOTHELIOMA (24)

This highly malignant neoplasm diffusely involves the pleura. Local extension and bloody pleural effusions are common. Patients with asbestos exposure have a high incidence of malignant mesothelioma. Peritoneal mesotheliomas have also been reported.

Laboratory—Anemia is common.

Chest Radiograph—Pleural based lesions with pleural effusion confined to the area of the patient's chest pain are the most characteristic findings.

Arterial Blood Gases—Hypoxemia is common.

Pulmonary Function Tests—Lung volumes are normal or decreased; flow rates are normal; DLCO is normal.

Miscellaneous—An increase in pleural fluid hyaluronic acid levels is diagnostic of this disease. Open lung biopsy is often needed to establish the diagnosis.[20,21]

BRONCHIAL ADENOMAS (25)

These are slow-growing intrabronchial lesions with three distinctive pathological classifications: bronchial carcinoids, cylindromas, and mucoepidermoid tumors. Although usually locally invasive, metastases to regional lymph nodes, liver, and bone have been reported.

Laboratory—No characteristic findings.

Chest Radiograph—Peripheral nodules and post-obstructive atelectasis or pneumonia are common.

Electrocardiogram—Normal.

Arterial Blood Gases—Hypoxemia may be present.

Pulmonary Function Tests—No characteristic pattern.

Miscellaneous—A very small percentage of patients with carcinoid tumors may exhibit the carcinoid syndrome (e.g., wheezing and flushing). Elevated levels of plasma serotonin should be sought in this condition.[22]

BACTERIAL, MYCOPLASMAL, AND RICKETTSIAL PNEUMONIAS (26)

Bacterial pneumonias can be arbitrarily classified as gram-negative or gram-positive by Gram stain; aerobic or anaerobic; lobar or bronchopneumonic; and localized or diffuse. These classifications are not mutually exclusive. Streptococcus pneumoniae (pneumococcal) pneumonias are still the most common bacterial pneumonias. Staphylococcal and gram-negative organisms cause pneumonias in hospitalized patients and immunocompromised hosts.

Mycoplasmas are the smallest free-living organisms, and they share a number of properties common to bacteria. The mycoplasmas can cause non-specific urethritis and bullous myringitis in addition to pneumonia.

Rickettsial pneumonias are associated with multisystem organ involvement due to a diffuse vasculitis. Rickettsiae are very small gram-negative bacteria. The most common diseases affecting the lungs are Rocky Mountain spotted fever and Q fever.

> Laboratory—In bacterial pneumonias, leukocytosis with a "shift to the left" (e.g., immature forms) is common. Leukopenia is a poor prognostic sign; hyponatremia is common. Sputum Gram stains and cultures may identify the offending organisms. Cold agglutinins are found in many patients with mycoplasmal pneumonias.
>
> Chest Radiograph—A variety of chest radiograph appearances are common and depend on the specific cause of the pneumonia.
>
> Electrocardiogram—Usually normal. Pneumonias that abut against the pericardium may cause transient atrial fibrillation and flutter.
>
> Arterial Blood Gases—Hypoxemia is common. In a small percentage of patients, respiratory failure is evidenced by hypercapnea.
>
> Pulmonary Function Tests—Clinically not helpful.[23]

VIRAL PNEUMONIAS (27)

Viral pneumonias are caused by a variety of viral agents and are usually associated with a high morbidity (e.g., time lost from work) but with a low mortality. Epidemics of influenzal viral pneumonia associated with a high mortality rate for both the young and the elderly are the exception to this rule.

> Laboratory—Usually normal.
>
> Chest Radiograph—Patchy or diffuse interstitial infiltrates are common.
>
> Electrocardiogram—Normal.
>
> Arterial Blood Gases—Hypoxemia is common.
>
> Pulmonary Function Tests—Not helpful.[24]

LUNG ABSCESSES (28)

This is a suppurative pulmonary infection causing destruction of lung parenchyma with formation of a cavity or cavities with air fluid levels. The lung destruction is due to the necrotizing character of the specific agent involved.

Laboratory—Anemia and leukocytosis are common. Sputum Gram stain will often identify the offending organisms.

Chest Radiograph—Small, multiple, and large single cavities (e.g., air fluid levels), often associated with pleural effusions, are characteristic.

Electrocardiogram—Normal.

Arterial Blood Gases—Hypoxemia is common.

Pulmonary Function Tests—Not helpful.[25,26]

PULMONARY TUBERCULOSIS (29)

This chronic infection caused by *Mycobacterium tuberculosis* is not limited to the lungs, but can affect bones, meninges, gastrointestinal tract, and genitourinary tract. The two forms of pulmonary tuberculosis are primary infection and reactivation. Patients at risk are those who are postgastrectomy, immunosuppressed, taking high-dose corticosteroids, pregnant, alcoholic, or with chronic renal failure.

Laboratory—The anemia of chronic disease is common. Leukocyte counts are variable. Sputum smears with the Ziehl–Neelsen stain reveal acid-fast organisms in patients with active cavitary disease or extensive pneumonia.

Chest Radiograph—A wide variety of patterns have been described, the most common being upper lobe, posterior infiltrates, and cavities with or without pleural effusions. Atypical presentations are common.

Arterial Blood Gases—Hypoxemia is common.

Electrocardiogram—Usually normal.

Pulmonary Function Tests—Not helpful.

Miscellaneous—Sputum specimens should be cultured to identify the organisms. Pleura cultures and biopsies may be helpful in patients with pleural effusions. If there is any suspicion of meningitis, urethritis, arthritis, and so on, the appropriate body fluid should be obtained and cultured for acid-fast organisms.[27]

ATYPICAL TUBERCULOSIS (30)

These ubiquitous mycobacteria are opportunistic in nature and found in soil, water, and milk. There is no evidence for human-to-human transmission. Clinically, pathologically, and radiologically, they produce a disease similar to tuberculosis. Many patients who develop atypical mycobacterial infections have underlying emphysema, chronic bronchitis, or bronchiectasis.

> *Laboratory*—Anemia is common. Sputum examination reveals acid-fast organisms and the sputum cultures aid in identification.
> *Chest Radiograph*—Similar to tuberculosis.
> *Electrocardiogram*—Usually normal.
> *Arterial Blood Gases*—Hypoxemia is common.
> *Pulmonary Function Tests*—Not helpful.[28,29]

ACTINOMYCES AND *NOCARDIA* (31)

Actinomycoses is a chronic systemic disease caused by *Actinomyces isrealii*, which is a pleomorphic, rod-shaped bacteria appearing in tissue as granules. These organisms are part of the normal mouth flora.

Nocardiosis is an acute or chronic suppurative infection usually caused by *Nocardia asteroides*, which are aerobic higher bacteria with branching, weakly gram-positive and acid-fast hyphae less than 1 μ wide. *Nocardia* organisms are found in soil and are usually saprophytic. The portal of entry is through the lungs.

> *Laboratory*—Anemia and leukocytosis are common. The organisms can be identified using appropriate sputum smears and cultures.
> *Chest Radiograph*—Single or multiple nodules and pleural effusions are common. *Actinomyces*, in contrast to *Nocardia*, forms sinus tracts through and into the thoracic wall.
> *Electrocardiogram*—Usually normal.
> *Arterial Blood Gases*—Hypoxemia is common.
> *Pulmonary Function Tests*—Not helpful.
> *Miscellaneous*—*Nocardia* has a propensity to spread to the brain causing metastatic abscesses.[30,31]

MYCOSES (32)

This group of systemic diseases includes histoplasmosis, coccidioidomycoses, blastomycosis, cryptococcosis, sporotrichosis, mucormycosis, aspergillosis, and candidiasis. Each organism causes a specific disease and is found in endemic areas, except for mucormycosis and aspergillosis, which are ubiquitous.

> *Laboratory*—Anemia and mild leukocytosis are common in all of these diseases. Sputum smear and cultures help identify the organisms.

Chest Radiograph—The radiologic findings depend on the specific disease and its stage. For example, in acute histoplasmosis, pulmonary infiltrates with hilar adenopathy are common; in chronic stages of this disease, cavities are characteristic. In patients with chronic coccidioidomycosis, thin-walled multiple cavities are common. Blastomycosis can cause both infiltrative parenchymal involvement and pleural effusions. Disseminated mucormycosis and aspergillosis cause a pulmonary infarction type pattern.

Electrocardiogram—Usually normal.

Arterial Blood Gases—Hypoxemia is common.

Pulmonary Function Tests—Not helpful.[31]

ASPIRATION LUNG DISEASES (33)

This disease can be caused by the aspiration of acid or neutral gastric content, nasopharyngeal flora, fresh or salt water, other liquids, and solid foreign bodies. Certain conditions predispose to aspiration, including altered states of consciousness, anesthesia, esophageal motility disorders, gastric reflux, tracheostomy, nasogastric tube placement, swallowing dysfunction, cardiac resuscitation, and general debilitation.

Laboratory—Leukocytosis is common.

Chest Radiograph—Depends on the type and extent of aspiration; may vary from normal to single, localized infiltrates to bilateral, diffuse infiltrates consistent with the adult respiratory distress syndrome (ARDS).

Electrocardiogram—Not helpful.

Arterial Blood Gases—Hypoxemia and hypocapnea are common. Hypercapnea may occur in patients with diffuse aspiration pneumonia.

Pulmonary Function Tests—Not helpful.[32]

PULMONARY ALVEOLAR PROTEINOSIS (34)

This is a disease of unknown etiology characterized by chronic and progressive alveolar filling with a proteinaceous, PAS-positive, and lipid-rich granular material felt to be derived from surfactant and cellular debris. For some reason, these patients are prone to colonization or infection with organisms such as *Nocardia*.

Laboratory—An elevated serum lactate dehydrogenase is common.

Chest Radiograph—Bilateral, diffuse "ground glass" infiltrates involving the perihilar region and mimicking pulmonary edema are characteristic.

Electrocardiogram—Normal.

Arterial and Blood Gases—Hypoxemia and hypocapnea are common. Hypoxemia is poorly responsive to elevated levels of FIO_2.

Pulmonary Function Tests—Lung volumes are decreased; flow rates are normal; DLCO is low.[33]

WEGENER'S GRANULOMATOSIS, ITS VARIANTS, AND OTHER VASCULITIDES (35)

Wegener's granulomatosis is a form of granulomatous vasculitis characterized by granuloma formation in addition to vascular inflammation. Wegener's classically consists of necrotizing granulomatous vasculitis of the upper and lower respiratory tracts, focal glomerulonephritis, and some degree of disseminated vasculitis. In addition, there are limited forms of Wegener's confined to the lungs and skin. Lymphomatoid granulomatosis, Churg–Strauss syndrome, necrotizing sarcoid granulomatosis, and bronchocentric granulomatosis comprise the remainder of these diseases.

Laboratory—Anemia and an active urinary sediment are common. Leukocytosis may be present.

Chest Radiograph—A variety of presentations are common. Parenchymal nodular densities with or without pleural effusions are characteristic.

Electrocardiogram—Usually normal.

Arterial Blood Gases—Hypoxemia is common.

Pulmonary Function Tests—Not helpful.

Miscellaneous—Biopsy of nasal or upper airway granulomas may establish diagnosis in Wegener's granulomatosis. Lung, skin, and kidney biopsies may be helpful.[34]

SLEEP APNEA AND CENTRAL HYPOVENTILATION SYNDROMES (36)

Apnea is defined as cessation of mouth air flow for 10-sec to 15-sec periods, occurring more than 30 times in an 8-hour sleep period. The apneas may be classified as obstructive or central in type. In obstructive apneas, posterior pharyngeal obstruction is associated with continued and labored thoracic movement. In central apneas, air flow and chest wall movement cease simultaneously. A combination of obstructive and central sleep apnea is also common.

Central hypoventilation is a disease of unknown etiology in which the patient hypoventilates during sleep and has depressed response to inhaled carbon dioxide. A similar disorder may follow high spinal cord or brainstem surgery. Apnea ensues when the patient falls asleep and sudden death is common. This syndrome is called *Ondine's curse.*

Laboratory—Polycythemia is common secondary to chronic hypoxemia.

Chest Radiograph—Usually normal.

Electrocardiogram—Normal or consistent with cor pulmonale.

Arterial Blood Gases—Daytime arterial blood gases may be normal during the early stage; however, nighttime blood gases reveal hypoxemia and eventually hypercapnea. These abnormalities may become persistent and be present during the day.

Pulmonary Function Tests—Usually normal, although in obese patients with the sleep apnea syndrome, lung volumes are decreased.

Miscellaneous—A history of snoring, daytime somnolence, change of personality, and weight gain are common in obstructive sleep apnea syndromes. Polysomnographic tracing will establish the diagnosis.[35,36]

REFERENCES

1. Hugh–Jones P, Whimster W: The etiology management of disabling emphysema. In Murray J (ed): Lung Disease: State of the Art, 1977–1978, pp 125–160. New York, American Lung Association, 1979
2. Hodgkins JE (ed): Chronic Obstructive Pulmonary Disease: Current Concepts and Diagnosis and Comprehensive Care, pp 1–32. Park Ridge, IL, American College of Chest Physicians, 1979
3. Williams MH: The nature of asthma: Definition and natural history. Semin Respir Med 1:283, 1980
4. Bolman RM, Wolfe WG: Bronchiectasis and bronchopulmonary sequestration. Surg Clin North Am 60:867–881, 1980
5. Holsclaw DS: Cystic Fibrosis: Overview and pulmonary aspects in young adults. Clin Chest Med 1:407–422, 1980
6. Kryger MH, Acres JC: Upper airway obstruction. Chest 80:207–211, 1981
7. Hunninghake GW, Faci AS: Pulmonary involvement in the collagen vascular diseases. In Murray J (ed): Lung Diseases—State of the Art, 1978–1979, pp 83–116. New York, American Lung Association, 1980

8. Mitchell DN, Scaddings JG: Sarcoidosis. Am Rev Respir Dis 110:774–802, 1974
9. Brigham K: Pulmonary edema—Cardiac and noncardiac Am J Surg 138:361, 1979
10. Bergofsky EH: Respiratory failure and disorders of thoracic cage. In Murray J (ed): Lung Disease—State of the Art, 1978–1979, pp 347–374. New York, American Lung Association, 1980
11. Brooks SM, Lockey JE, Harber P (eds): Occupational Lung Diseases (1). Clinics in Chest Medicine, Vol. 2, pp 169–288. Philadelphia, WB Saunders, 1981
12. Roberts RC, Moore VL: Immunopathogenesis of hypersensitivity pneumonitis. In Murray J (ed): Lung Disease—State of the Art, 1977–1978, pp 213–228. New York, American Lung Association, 1979
13. Morgan PGM, Turner-Warwick M: Pulmonary hemosiderosis and pulmonary hemorrhage. Br J Dis Chest 75:225–242, 1981
14. Davidson AR: Eosinophilic granuloma of the lung. Br J Chest Dis 70:125–127, 1976
15. Moser KM: Pulmonary embolism. In Murray J (ed): Lung Disease—State of the Art, 1976–1977, pp 1–24. New York, American Lung Association, 1978
16. Fishman AP: Chronic cor pulmonale. In Murray J (ed): Lung Disease—State of the Art, 1976–1977, pp 355–374. New York, American Lung Association, 1978
17. Young RC, Jr, Castro O, Baxter RP et al: The lung in sickle cell disease: A clinical overview of common vascular infections and other problems. J Natl Med Asso 73:19–26, 1981
18. Cohen MH: Natural history of lung carcinoma. Clin Chest Dis 3:229–241, 1982
19. Lillington GA: Pulmonary nodules: Solitary and multiple. Clin Chest Dis 3:361–367, 1982
20. Chahinian AP, Pajak TF, Holland JF et al: Diffuse malignant mesothelioma. Prospective evaluation of 69 patients. Ann Intern Med 96:746–755, 1982
21. Craighead JE, Mossman BT: The pathogenesis of asbestos association diseases. N Engl J Med 306:1446–1455, 1982
22. Lawson RN, Ramanathan L, Hurley G et al: Bronchial adenoma: Review of an 18 year experience at the Brompton Hospital. Thorax 31:245, 1976
23. Frame PT: Acute infectious pneumonia in the adult. Basics Respir Dis 10:1–8, 1982
24. Jackson GG, Kilbourne ED: Viral infections of the respiratory tract. In Beson PB, McDermott W, Wyngaarden JB (eds): Cecil's Textbook of Medicine 15th ed, pp 230–246. Philadelphia, WB Saunders, 1979
25. Alexander JC, Wolfe WG: Lung abscess and empyema of the thorax. Surg Clin North Am 60:835–849, 1980
26. Schachter EN: Supprative lung diseases: Old problems revisited. Clin Chest Med 1:41–50, 1981
27. Sted WW, Dutt AK: Tuberculosis. Clin Chest Dis 1:165–263, 1980
28. Rosenzweig DY: Atypical "mycobacterioses." Clin Chest Med 1:273–284, 1980
29. Wolinsky E: Nontuberculous mycobacteria and associated diseases. In Murray J (ed): Lung Disease—State of the Art, 1978–1979, pp 1–53. New York, American Lung Association, 1980
30. Weese WC, Smith IM: A study of 57 cases of actinomycosis over a 36-year period. Arch Intern Med 135:1562, 1975
31. Hammon JW, Frayer RL: Surgical management of fungal diseases of the chest. Surg Clin North Am 60:897–912, 1980
32. Cooper KR, Fairman RP, Glauser FL: Current issues in pulmonary acid aspiration therapy. ER Reports 1:115–118, 1980
33. Costello JF, Moriarty DC, Branthwante MA et al: Diagnosis and management of alveolar proteinosis: The role of electron microscopy. Thorax 30:121–132, 1915
34. Edwards CW: Vasculitis and granulomatosis of the respiratory tract. Thorax 37:81–87, 1982
35. Reichel J: Primary alveolar hypoventilation. Clin Chest Med 1:119–124, 1980
36. Guilleninault C, Dement WC (eds): Sleep Apnea Syndromes, pp 1–12. New York, Allan R. Liss, 1978

INDEX

The letter f indicates a figure; the letter t represents tabular material.

Abscess, lung, 227–228
  breath and voice sounds in, 136
  chest pain in, 34
  clubbing in, 182
  cough in, 18
  crackles and wheezes in, 148
  cyanosis in, 198
  fever, chills, nightsweats in, 76
  hemoptysis in, 41
  percussion in, 159
  respiratory muscles in, 123
  sputum in, 26
  tachypnea in, 104
  weight loss in, 63
  wheezing in, 51
Accessory muscle use quantification, 114t
Actinomyces and *Nocardia*, 229
  altered mental status, headache, coma in, 57
  chest pain in, 34
  fever, chills, nightsweats in, 77
  percussion in, 159
  tachypnea in, 105
Adenoma, bronchial. See Bronchial adenoma
Adventitious lung sounds, 138–149
  in infectious lung disease, 148–149
  mechanisms of, 139f, 140–144, 141f–144f
  in obstructive lung disease, 145
  in pulmonary vascular disease, 147
  in restrictive lung disease, 146–147
  in specific pulmonary diseases, 144–149
  terminology in, 139
  in tumors of lung, pleura, mediastinum, 148
Airway diameter and lung volume, 44, 44f
Airway outlet, voluntary contraction of, 45
Airway tortuosity, 43
Altered mental status, headache, coma, 53–58
  in infectious lung disease, 57
  mechanisms of, 53–55
  in obstructive lung disease, 56
  in pulmonary vascular disease, 56
  in restrictive lung disease, 56
  specific pulmonary diseases and, 55–57
  symptoms of, 55
  in tumors of lung, pleura, mediastinum, 57
Alveolar proteinosis, 230–231
  breath and voice sounds in, 136
  crackles and wheezes in, 149
  fever in, 77
  tachypnea in, 105
Anemia
  cyanosis in, 193, 194f
  hemolysis-induced, 54
Angina pectoris, 29
Anorexia and weight loss, 59–65
  in carcinoma of lung, pleura, mediastinum, 63

  dietary factors in, 59
  in infectious lung disease, 63–64
  mechanisms of, 59–60
  in obstructive lung disease, 61–62
  in pulmonary vascular disease, 63
  in restrictive lung disease, 62–63
  in specific pulmonary disease, 61–64
Aortic dissection, 30–31
Articular pain, 80–81
Aspiration lung disease, 230
  breath and voice sounds in, 136
  cough in, 18
  crackles and wheezes in, 149
  cyanosis in, 198
  dyspnea in, 10
  fever, chills, nightsweats in, 77
  hoarseness and snoring in, 94
  percussion in, 159
  respiratory muscles in, 123
  sputum in, 26
  tachypnea in, 105
  wheezing in, 51
Asterixis, 183–188
  differential diagnosis of, 186
  mechanisms and definition of, 183–185, 184f
  patient characteristics in pulmonary disease with, 186–187
  pathophysiology of, 185
  in specific pulmonary diseases, 187–188
Asthma, 213
  altered mental status, headache, coma in, 56
  breath and voice sounds in, 123
  cardiac findings in, 167
  cough in, 15
  cyanosis in, 196
  dyspnea in, 6
  percussion in, 155
  respiratory muscles in, 120
  sputum in, 23
  tachypnea in, 101
  wheezing in, 48, 145

Body heat
  elimination of, 68–69
  sources of, 67
Body temperature
  central nervous system regulation of, 69, 70f
  diurnal, 67, 68f
  normal, 66–67
  regulation of, 67
Breath- and voice-generated sounds, 125–137
  abnormal, 130–131
  in infectious lung disease, 136
  mechanisms of, 126–127
  normal, 128–129, 129f
  in obstructive lung disease, 132–133
  in pulmonary vascular disease, 135